## Praise for *Sex and Y[...]*

"Stefanie Iris Weiss has created an experiential, dynamic, and completely new way to explore and heal our sexuality. This is not just a book; it's a portal into the way our bodies experience the seasons as they shift and change, using the archetypes of astrology. Weiss reminds us that pleasure is a force for healing ourselves, the people we love, and the Earth itself."

**Annie Sprinkle, PhD**
author of *The Explorer's Guide to Planet Orgasm* and
coauthor of *Assuming the Ecosexual Position*

"*Sex and Your Stars* skillfully intertwines the scientific and soulful aspects of eroticism and astrology. *Sex and Your Stars* introduces fresh perspectives, evokes new emotions, and encourages transformative practices through the lens of astrology. This work serves as a vital addition to the astrological canon, providing valuable insights that both inform and inspire without judgment. A compelling read, it offers essential support in reclaiming pleasures and embracing a more vibrant and fully alive existence."

**Colin Bedell**
author of *A Little Bit of Astrology* and *Queer Cosmos*

"*Sex and Your Stars* is a novel approach to solving sexual dilemmas using the language of astrology. The book shows us how to smash shame, engage with our desires, and choose to prioritize pleasure. A groundbreaking book that should be on the shelves of all sexuality professionals, it introduces innovative tools to help us understand and heal our bodies (and our souls), setting the stage for erotic empowerment and connection."

**Patti Britton, PhD**
founder of Sex Coach U and author of *The Art of Sex Coaching*

"Many of us are looking for ways to understand ourselves better. We want to learn more about our sexual and romantic needs, what we require from a partner in order to feel safe and fulfilled, and how to express our emotions in a healthy manner. We want to be the best partner we can be to the person(s) we love, but we also don't want to sacrifice too much of ourselves. We want a different approach to our analysis and introspection. *Sex and Your Stars* offers just that: a different way of thinking, a different set of questions, and a different way to view ourselves, our relationships, and the world. It's a must-read for the spiritual soul who's been feeling a little stuck."

**Zachary Zane**

author of *Boyslut*

"Even if you don't happen to be a keen believer in astrology, *Sex and Your Stars* is a wise book packed with profound insights, using the frame of our unique erotic archetype as a creative way to explore ourselves as sexual beings. As a sexologist, Ms. Weiss gets it, as evidenced by this quote: 'Learning what feels good may seem like it should be a "natural" process, but often, it's buried in layers of shame and societal ideas of what we're "supposed" to look and feel like, no matter our sexual or gender identity, race, ability, age, or body type.' *Sex and Your Stars* can help the reader engage with enthusiasm and playfulness in the quest to restore sexual pleasure as a healing force."

**Nan Wise, PhD**

author of *Why Good Sex Matters*

"Stefanie Iris Weiss has combined her considerable talents as a certified clinical sexologist and professional astrologer to help us forge our own unique path to sexual liberation. The journey to sexual sovereignty begins with shedding shame and finding pleasure in our own bodies. *Sex and Your Stars* shows us how to use astrological archetypes to move toward erotic embodiment, making space for deep intimacy, transcendent passion, and secure bonds with our lover(s). A delightful read and an important contribution to both astrology and sexology."

**Barbara Carrellas**

author of *Urban Tantra*

"Reading Stefanie Iris Weiss's *Sex and Your Stars* is orgasmic in just the way she wants it to be—starting in your brain. As a sexologist and an astrologer, Weiss draws on her expertise, experience, and transformative stories from her client files with concrete steps to move readers past any shame to become more of their true erotic selves. Although you can pick it up and read for your Sun, Moon, or rising sign, you'll gain much more from reading through the complete book. We have all twelve zodiac signs along with three archetypes of desire (Venus, Mars, and Black Moon Lilith) within us, and Weiss shows us how to bring our whole chart alive in our bodies with a lively and loving touch."

**Sam Reynolds**

astrology teacher and consultant

"Combining her decades of experience in both astrology and sexology, Stefanie Iris Weiss has written an illuminating and practical guidebook on how to live a life infused with more pleasure, sensuality, and erotic empowerment. Not only is *Sex and Your Stars* a stellar treasure for anyone wanting to more fully embrace and align with their passions and desires, but I can see it being an essential resource for astrologers looking for additional ways to help their clients live deeply meaningful and enriching lives."

**Stephanie Gailing**

author of *The Complete Guide to Living by the Moon*

# Sex
## AND YOUR
# Stars

## Also by Stefanie Iris Weiss

*Eco-Sex: Go Green Between the Sheets and Make Your Love Life Sustainable* (Crown Publishing)

*Spirit Animals: Unlocking the Secrets of Our Animal Companions* (Chronicle Books)

*Fate of Your Date: Divination for Dating, Mating, and Relating* (Chronicle Books)

*Surviving Saturn's Return: Overcoming the Most Tumultuous Time of Your Life* (McGraw-Hill)

# Sex
## AND YOUR
# Stars

## A Sexologist's Guide to the
## Erotic Energy of the Zodiac

## Stefanie Iris Weiss

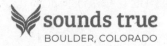
sounds true
BOULDER, COLORADO

Sounds True
Boulder, CO

This book is not intended as a substitute for the medical recommendations of
physicians, mental health professionals, or other health-care providers. Rather, it is
intended to offer information to help the reader cooperate with physicians, mental
health professionals, and health-care providers in a mutual quest for optimal well-
being. We advise readers to carefully review and understand the ideas presented and
to seek the advice of a qualified professional before attempting to use them.

Some names and identifying details have been changed to protect the privacy of
individuals.

Published 2024

Cover design by Jennifer Miles
Book design by Meredith Jarrett

Printed in the United States of America

BK06938

Library of Congress Cataloging-in-Publication Data

Names: Weiss, Stefanie Iris, author.
Title: Sex and your stars : a sexologist's guide to the erotic energy of the zodiac /
    Stefanie Iris Weiss.
Description: Boulder, CO : Sounds True, 2024. | Includes bibliographical
    references and index.
Identifiers: LCCN 2023051127 (print) | LCCN 2023051128 (ebook)
    | ISBN 9781649632630 (trade paperback) | ISBN
    9781649632647 (ebook)
Subjects: LCSH: Astrology and sex. | Astrology.
Classification: LCC BF1729.S4 W45 2024  (print) | LCC
    BF1729.S4  (ebook) | DDC 133.5/83067--dc23/
    eng/20240308
LC record available at https://lccn.loc.gov/2023051127
LC ebook record available at https://lccn.loc.gov/2023051128

FSC
www.fsc.org
MIX
Paper | Supporting
responsible forestry
FSC® C103098

*For my mom, who taught me to love fully and freely.*

# Contents

# Introduction

## Why Explore the Sex in Our Stars?

Sex energy and creative energy are parts of the same
life force that draws us to it like the warmth of a
summer sun or the light of a full moon.

**Betty Dodson**

*Sex for One: The Joy of Selfloving*

As above, so below.

**Astrological Proverb**

Humans have looked to the stars for guidance since we emerged from the primordial muck, and we've probably wrestled with our sexual desires for just as long. From the Babylonians to the Chinese, the Hellenistic, Islamicate, Mayan, and Vedic branches, to the Greeks and Romans, the astrologers of the European Renaissance, and finally to our own twenty-first-century star-whisperers making viral internet memes, astrology has been a lens for our relationships and sensual longings since the beginning of time.[1]

As we love and long to be loved, desire and long to be desired, connect and long to be connected, we often seek to understand both *why* and *how*. Poets, philosophers, and songwriters might give us some insight, but astrology, I've learned, can get us down into the deep, dirty, and decisive details.

This ancient art shows us how our natal chart (the planetary map astrologers draw based on a person's date, time, and place of birth) works as the cosmic fingerprint of our psyche. This can provide surprisingly accurate and penetrating insights into the question of when, how, and why we want what we want across our lifetimes and, helpfully, across the astrological seasons of each year.

Questions I often hear from astrology and clinical sexology clients tend to go something along these lines: "How can I live my richest, most fulfilled life sexually, relationally, and creatively?" If we're attracted to someone, experience pangs of romantic love, or want to be touched in a particular way, we might ask ourselves: Where did this longing come from? When we fantasize and masturbate, we may wonder why certain scenes play through our minds and turn us on. When we connect to another human deeply but nonsexually, we might similarly ask: Why are my feelings platonic? And central to working through all of this, when we experience shame about our desires or sexual experiences, we might ask ourselves: Is this my upbringing, my culture, my genetics, or is there something more to deconstruct?

## The Shadow-Banning of Astrology and Sexuality Through History

Sexology is the scientific study of human sexuality, interests, and behaviors. Long before the formal field of scientific sexology existed as a discipline, and in eras and within cultures where exploration of sexuality was forced into hiding, astrology was often there, giving us coded answers to our most secret, subversive questions. Like witchcraft and other occult practices, astrology has also been periodically forced underground; but like our natural, normal human desires, it persists.

Even in the third decade of the new millennium, where the future is now, some archconservative movements condemn astrology as the work of the devil. For me, both astrology and sexology (an inherently inclusive, queer-coded field) are threats to the heteropatriarchy and other systemic forms of oppression. What I love about both professions is that they aim to set individuals free to make their own choices and to be rulers of their own fates and desires—at least the way I practice them.

This book is about sexual self-knowledge and pleasure, and I can't let it go unsaid: we must fight the fascist forces coming for the rights of the most marginalized people in our society, because everyone's sexuality is sacred, not shameful.

## The Origins of Sexology

The formal academic discipline of sexology offers insight, depth, and peer-reviewed research when you're seeking counsel about your own sexuality or have questions about your sexual relationships. Sexology emerged as an academic discipline around the turn of the twentieth century, and over the last hundred-plus years, trailblazers from Alfred Kinsey (father of the Kinsey Scale) to Betty Dodson (groundbreaking proponent of women's masturbation) to Shere Hite (pioneering clitoris advocate) to my mentor, Dr. Patti Britton (the fabulous mother of sex coaching), have grappled with the science of sexuality, healing our intimate lives in the process.

If you're worried about some aspect of your sexuality or are seeking enhanced pleasure, the guidance of a certified clinical sexologist, trained sex coach, or sex therapist can be invaluable. Books and other self-enrichment tools are fantastic adjuncts for any journey to sexual sovereignty, but nothing can replace this expert professional context when you're in acute distress about a sexual matter. The resources section in this book includes information about how to find someone to work with, if you're ready for that step.

This book relies on research and time-tested tools that sexologists and sex coaches use in their practices, and also incorporates my training and professional work as a certified clinical sexologist and ongoing training in somatic sexology, not to mention my decade as a sex writer, reading and researching the literature on this juicy, fascinating topic.

From low libido to erectile dysfunction to mismatched desire to communication breakdowns to dating deficits, so much of what I see in my practice can be addressed when we work through the shame we retain about our sexuality from childhood and regressive cultural tropes we continue to encounter as adults. Even the most progressive, liberal, erudite, and sexually experienced of us know what shame feels like. You might be surprised at how your seemingly uber-confident and sexually sophisticated friend really feels when they're naked and getting it on.

If you feel like you know less about sex than you'd like to or have experienced less of it, you're far from alone.

I can't begin to tell you how many self-defined libertines, sex party regulars, and owners of drawers full of the latest sex tech—those who've made exploring their sexuality into a personal quest—have come to me in search of answers about long-standing shame they can't quite purge. Exploring sexuality brings out our vulnerabilities; that's part of why it's such liberatory personal work. How have we achieved a breakthrough? In many cases, by diving into their astrology charts.

## Combatting Sexual Impostor Syndrome with Astrology

One of my favorite sex therapists and authors, Yana Tallon-Hicks, coined the phrase "sexual imposter syndrome" in her book *Hot and Unbothered: How to Think About, Talk About, and Have the Sex You Really Want*. Like the kind of impostor syndrome we might experience when we're at a new job or just don't believe we deserve success, this phrase succinctly summarizes what we may feel when we try to show up in our sex lives without having worked through our shame.

Understanding your unique astrology archetype can give you a kind of cheat sheet for the way that shame might appear in your life—and in your sex life. We can usually find the roots of our sexual imposter syndrome in our charts, the same way we can find our childhood experiences, parenting, and relationship patterns in our charts. *Sex and Your Stars* will help you explore and expunge the shame you're holding onto, no matter where you are in your sexual journey.

Something I find myself saying to clients, repeating in workshops, and writing over, and over, and over again: *sex always begins with your relationship to your own body*. Learning what feels good may seem like it should be a "natural" process, but often, it's buried in layers of shame and societal ideas of what we're "supposed" to look and feel like, no matter our sexual or gender identity, race, ability, age, or body type.

The truth is that a healthy relationship to pleasure and embodiment (or the mind/body connection) takes work. Our nervous systems are very often compromised by trauma, either personal or collective. Sometimes the process of letting ourselves melt into sensation feels like a soft unpeeling, but sometimes it feels like an unbearable chiseling. Using our astrological charts as a guide can help us lean into the softer side of the pleasure/embodiment continuum.

## Sexual Astrology: A Way to See into the Erotic Self

If we understand astrology to be a system of personality archetypes and their psychological correspondences, this practice can bring enormous depth to our understanding of the erotic self. Astrologers define *archetypes* in different ways, but I love Steven Forrest's definition from the glossary of his book *The Inner Sky*. He says an archetype is "a fundamental image held collectively and universally in human consciousness; the mythic raw material out of which individual identity is synthesized." Certainly not all people of the same Sun sign or other planetary placements embody all the layers of a particular archetype. But often, the ones that apply to you and your life will resonate so powerfully that the first time you learn about them, you might get the chills or laugh at the spot-on accuracy of it all.

My version of *sexual astrology* takes the modern, scientifically rigorous field of sexology and marries it to the ancient, perennial, and complex art of astrology. In my work with clients, I call this an *Erotic Energy Mapping* session, during which I share the many ways the natal chart illuminates our sexual selves. Together, these two fields can supplement and heighten your understanding of human longings, attractions, relationship patterns, and sexual boundaries or concerns.

A significant benefit of layering astrological knowledge into your understanding of human sexuality is this: it can help to reduce some of the shame you carry about your desires. How? When you are better versed in the psychosexual patterns common to your astrology chart, you might stop blaming yourself for issues that come up repeatedly in your relationships, attraction patterns, or even in the way your body reacts to sexual stimuli. This provides a more immediate, instant portal into our sexuality, a subject that can be fraught. If you seek to better understand your own sexual urges, fetishes, blocks, and concerns, getting inside your natal chart can supplement and nourish that understanding, providing more pleasure.

Learning the basic astrological archetypes that may describe you, a long-term partner, casual hookup, or ex-lover you're not quite over can open vast landscapes of empathy and support that you can then extend to yourself and your beloved(s). Tapping into this astrological, erotic, and energetic matrix adds color and dimension to sex and relationships and has the power to unveil pleasure you've never accessed before. Knowing what might turn on, unlock, ease, and please us becomes a bit less loaded and a lot more fun.

For me, all astrology is a lived experience—and in the realm of sexual astrology, even more so. Understanding our sexual selves is a holistic experience, from our hearts to our minds to our erogenous zones (found all over the body) and genitals (although we can have plenty of sex that doesn't include our genitals). The aim of sexual astrology, as I understand and practice it, is to feel our charts in our bodies, rather than simply comprehending them intellectually or analyzing them from the proverbial psychoanalytic couch (although, trust me, I do plenty of this later in this book, too). The deeper we go into the archetypes of each sign and planet, the more we can feel them moving through us and recognize when an emotion, sensation, or desire invokes our natal chart or a current transit (how the orbiting planets interact with the natal chart). Making astrology into a lived experience can mean tracking the lunar cycles, tracking your menstrual cycles as they correspond to the lunar cycles, planting by the Moon, using herbs and foods that correspond to particular planets in your chart to strengthen them, observing the planets with a telescope, going out under the stars on clear nights to simply drink in their majesty, or masturbating or having sex when the planets interact with one of your sensitive natal planets. When you meet someone who, for no discernable reason, fires up your loins and later find out that their chart's Venus is in the same sign as your Mars—one of many possible examples of *sexual synastry* (a way of putting people's charts together to see how the planets "talk" to one another)—that's making astrology into a lived experience, too.

## My Journey to Astrology and Sexology

Before I was a certified clinical sexologist or an astrologer, I was just a young writer trying to find my way; writing is what brought me to both professions. Astrology is a language of time-keeping, and I grew attracted to it, in part, because of its rich, riveting mythology and poetry. If you find yourself keeping company with astrologers, don't be shocked about the ubiquity of the poetry-to-astrology pipeline—it's a THING. A lot of people find their way to astrology through horoscopes—I found my way to it through the power of myth and metaphor. But don't get me wrong—I have written a LOT of horoscopes, and done well, they have great value. I began practicing astrology professionally around the year 2000 and began writing about sexuality around 2010. Writing about sex is something that I always wanted to do—this trait is in my chart!

Long before I was widely known as a sexuality expert and years before I published *Eco-Sex*, my first book about sex, my astrology clients often asked me questions about their sex lives and secret desires, questions they told me they weren't comfortable asking other practitioners or even their therapists. I always welcomed these erotic deep dives, but for a long time, I wasn't sure why they sought *me* out for this. By the time I had a column called *Sexual Healing* for a now-defunct website called *EcoSalon*, later delving into New York's sexual underground in reported pieces for *Narratively* and *The Daily Dot*, it became more common for clients to find me through my sex writing and then say, "Oh wow, you're also an astrologer!" Or it would be the opposite—my astrology clients would see a sexuality piece I posted on social media and message me to ask if they could come in for a session explicitly about sexual concerns they were having.

I was lucky to be raised in a household where conversations about bodies and sex were frank and easy—any questions I had were answered in an inherently practical, straightforward, shame-free way by my mom, who was born and bred in the People's Republic of Brooklyn (where they don't have time for bullshit). My parents also owned a head shop called The Magic Cottage before I was born and briefly when I was a toddler, just so you can get a sense of my very-comfortable-with-human-bodies vibe.

When I was seven and saw a tampon on the bathroom sink, I asked what it was—and that led to my earliest conversation about reproduction and sex. We didn't use cutesy terms for body parts in my house: when I was three, I knew that my vagina was a vagina, not a "vajayjay" or "down there" (although it took until adulthood for me to learn the difference between a vagina and a vulva). My mom laughs when I tell her that she's the reason I became a sexologist, but there was a pretty clear pathway! This is all to say that before I formally began studying sexology, I was always comfortable and candid in astrology sessions when clients asked questions about intimacy issues, as comfortable as I've always been talking to my friends about sex. Once again, thanks, mom!

I began to blend sexuality into my astrological client work in the mid-aughts. My regular clients knew they could say something like "I'm not feeling turned on when my partner touches me" and get insight into a chart placement or transit without feeling weird or exposed. This, in part, is how I was able to build and refine the body of knowledge that informs the content of this book.

## How I Do Astrology

I'm a self-taught astrologer, and my early training (basically reading every book in print about astrology) and informal study with a few different mentors was in what we call "modern astrology," with an emphasis on evolutionary and psychological astrology. You might sometimes hear "modern astrology" used pejoratively, as there's been an online turf war between some people who study traditional astrology and those who came up as moderns. I steer clear of those wars. As traditional methods became more accessible in the last decade or so, I began to study those, too. Even though I'm a professional astrologer who has had thousands of clients, I'll be learning new techniques for the rest of my life: that's how vast the astrological pantheon is. As someone who draws from the deep wells of both psychological and traditional astrology, I'm out here wishing we could all get along.

In the last thirty years, but more definitively since the early 2010s, there has been an absolute sea change in the way many Americans understand and experience astrology (coinciding with Neptune's transit through Pisces, not so incidentally). Astrology went from being a subculture, something only your hippy-dippy or LA friends were into, to being everywhere, all the time. The *New Yorker*, the *New York Times*, and *The Atlantic* covered the astrology boom with serious, reported pieces in the year or two before the pandemic.

Two things happened in the last thirty years that have likely changed the course of astrology forever. The internet and apps gave millions of people instant access to their own charts, right at their fingertips— suddenly, everyone knew their rising sign. My best friend and astrology partner and I had spent hundreds of brunches speaking the language of astrology prior to this era in the early 2000s, casually dropping "I will probably see him again even though his Saturn is on my Moon" over coffee and omelets in New York City, getting intense "What, are you some kind of weirdo?" side-eye. Suddenly, we started hearing the people at the table next to us *using the same language*—and we knew something unprecedented was happening.

Many, if not most, astrologers who've come to the profession in the last fifteen years or so learned their craft as students of traditional astrology,[2] which differs in fundamental ways from modern astrology, the astrological language I was first introduced to in the nineties. For example, as Uranus, Neptune, and Pluto were not yet discovered when the Greeks and Egyptians developed their techniques, these planets are not considered by those who exclusively practice traditional astrology. There are excellent arguments to be made for both ways of doing astrology, or of weaving them together like I do (and dozens of other ways of doing it, like Sidereal astrology, a different system based on the fixed stars), and this is not the place to historicize the debate between modern and traditional astrologers. However, I mention all of this so you know where I'm coming from as an astrologer—which is to say that I use various analyses and techniques, sometimes in one session.

One important part of my methodology is key to this book: I practice astrology using the tropical zodiac, so my relationship to the zodiac and understanding of the signs is based on the seasons. Tropical astrology, practiced by most Western astrologers, considers the position of the Sun in relationship to the vernal equinox—the first day of spring, and in our parlance, zero degrees of Aries. Sidereal astrology considers the *precession* of the equinoxes, so the dates of each zodiac season continue to change over time. Vedic astrology, which uses the Sidereal system, originated in India some five thousand years ago, is still widely practiced there, and is increasingly popular among Western practitioners as well. Even Sidereal enthusiasts, however, can gain insights from *Sex and Your Stars*, because the astrological sign archetypes are present across disciplines. If you're interested in learning more about Sidereal astrology, the resources section offers some options.

In short, my concept of the zodiac is generated by the equinoxes and solstices that divide the year and is set up along the ecliptic of twelve signs through which the Sun passes. That's how we get Aries through Pisces, or Aries season through Pisces season. Note that even in the Southern Hemisphere, where the seasons are reversed, most Western astrologers rely on the tropical zodiac, so Aries season would always begin at the vernal equinox, when the amount of day and night is the same in both hemispheres.

## Sun Signs and Sexuality

The Sun is the heart of your astrology chart: this is the first (and often only) thing that most people know about their natal charts, mainly because it's easy and accessible information. When people ask you, "What's your sign?" what they're really asking is, "What's your Sun sign?"

We all revolve around our Sun, so it is near and dear to us. And yes, this book is called *Sex and Your Stars*, but we only have one star in this sweet little solar system of ours. As I mentioned, since astrology has become more popular and prominent, many people, especially

Millennials and Gen Z (or anyone who lives on the internet), are conversant with the meaning of the Sun, Moon, and rising sign—what astrologers call the "big three." We can also thank eminent astrologer Chani Nicholas, author of *You Were Born for This*, for teaching the broader public about their big three. Knowing your rising sign is VERY valuable, especially when you're hoping to understand your current transits or to know where the planets live in your chart.

When we are the subjects of our own analysis, the Sun stands out as a powerful tool for self-knowledge. Think of it this way—it's the only celestial body that always creates a shadow. The Sun has gotten something of a bad rap in astrology in recent years, and I aim to create a new space for us to swing the pendulum once again toward loving and exploring our Sun signs' rich potential and inherent vitality—especially when it comes to understanding our sexual selves.

We often only know a person's birthday or birth month, and thus their Sun sign. If you meet someone at a bar or a dinner party and don't feel like whipping out your handy astrology app, you're limited to a straightforward Sun sign analysis—yet this is a lot more valuable than you might think, so I encourage you to spend some time with it.

The Sun, in some ways, is the main character of the natal chart: the orb that shines brightest, hottest, and strongest of all the other planets. Note that the Sun and Moon are not actually planets: in astrology, we call them the "lights" or "luminaries"—because they are the celestial bodies that bring us light.[3]

Solar deities have been worshipped across civilizations from time immemorial as life-givers and sustainers. Without the Sun, we cannot grow and thrive—or eat, for that matter. Our mitochondria depend upon it. In our charts, the Sun is our survival instinct and our basic energetic imprint. Applying solar principles to modern Western psychology (more specifically, analytical psychology), the Sun is our ego and our conscious mind. This can translate to our will, our creative and erotic drives, our vitality and reason for being. Our soul longs to serve the mission of our Sun sign. As endlessly complex as a natal chart is, and there are thousands of permutations in each one, our Sun, in many ways, is what we aspire to become.

If the Sun is our ego, then it drives the brain, our largest sexual organ, to find its way in the world and weave together our relationships, as well as our relationship with the self. The interplay between our psychosexual behavior and our Sun sign is so very basic that once you read the first twelve chapters of this book, you may be astonished at how aptly they describe you and the people you know and love.

When we explore the complexities of eros, a concept I'll get into shortly, Sun sign analysis serves us well. Yes, understanding your astrosexual self is far more complicated than your Sun sign alone. But if the Sun is the heart of our natal fingerprint, it shines its revealing and singular light on the rest of our horoscope. When we want to understand what drives our erotic nature, the Sun shows us where to find the heat. A more complete sexual examination of our psyche, desire nature, kinks, and attractions might consider the houses of the natal chart, the Moon, the placement of Venus and Mars and their mathematical relationship to the Sun and other planets, and Black Moon Lilith (the Moon's apogee). Most of this is within the purview of the book you have in your hot little hands. Because the Moon is so well covered by other great books, I discuss it where it's relevant, especially in the Cancer chapter, but I haven't devoted a whole chapter to it. Instead, I've included some of my favorite books on this topic in the resources section.

If you want the *whole* package and the deeper context that comes with knowing your entire natal chart, you'll need to dial up your friendly neighborhood astrologer, because it's too complex for any single text. But this book can get you far, especially if you choose to use it across the astrological seasons.

## A Note on Rising Signs

The Aries through Pisces chapters of *Sex and Your Stars* are designed to speak to the erotic energy inherent in our Sun signs and the seasons that accompany them each year. However, if you *do* know your own or another person's rising sign, the chapters that correspond to those signs are likely to resonate deeply as well, so read them too. Why? Because the rising sign is what we project outwardly to the world, and it's the most uniquely *you* part of your chart. It's also, importantly, very relevant to how we experience *transits* (the way the orbiting planets interact with our chart throughout our lives). Our rising sign is generally what others first experience and perceive about us when they meet us, and often, we first experience this part of our personality around the time of puberty or early adolescence, when we're figuring out what our peers' expectations are of us. This is also the time, notably, that hormones are surging through our body and weaving our ever-evolving sexuality.

The Sun, depending on where it is placed and its relative strength in the chart, may not be the dominant personality trait you see in yourself or that others perceive right away, and it might take some digging to reveal. Sometimes as people get older (after their Saturn Return at twenty-nine-and-a-half), they become more acquainted and comfortable with their Sun sign. Ideally, with maturity, growth, and experience, the Sun and rising sign find a healthy balance with one another, each secure in their role. In short, depending on the situation or life circumstance, you might find that your own or another person's rising sign chapter is a stronger match. Understanding the natal Sun as an instinctive and *aspirational* energy can simplify this.

Sun sign–based relationship astrology is the stuff of legend, going back to brilliant astrologer and writer Linda Goodman's *Love Signs,* published in the seventies—a book that helped popularize astrology as a tool to understand relationships and compatibility. We can do without the antiquated, oppressive gender stereotypes of that time, however. Unfortunately, these categories have persisted in some sexual and romantic compatibility astrology books even in recent years. Luckily, many younger astrologers are pushing the field to break free of these limiting ideas of human behavior and desire. I'm a Gen-Xer, but I'm totally here for this! The queering and decolonizing of astrology is thankfully moving forward full steam in the United States, but it can take some time for language inspired by Greek and Roman gods and goddesses to catch up with what our hearts know: that love is love. That said, for the purpose of clarity and simplicity, I may refer to classically masculine planets like Mars and Saturn as he/him and classically feminine planets like Venus and the Moon as she/her, and do the same for associated deities.

This book embraces sexual astrology for the *true* Age of Aquarius, that elusive era that people have talked about since the sixties, when we're all meant to come together as one. Now we have the opportunity to be wholly inclusive and embrace the LGBTQIA+ spectrum, including people of all intersecting gender, sex, sexual orientation, race, ability, and other identities. No matter how we identify, our astrology chart sets us free to truly know ourselves, to shed our shame, and to explore our erotic energy with others.

# 1

# Charting the Sex in Your Stars

## How to Use This Book

I can hear the sizzle of newborn stars, and know anything of
meaning, of the fierce magic emerging here. I am witness to flexible
eternity, the evolving past, and I know we will live forever, as dust
or breath in the face of stars, in the shifting pattern of winds.

**Joy Harjo**

*Secrets from the Center of the World, Volume 17*

Your journey through *Sex and Your Stars* can be as unique as your
birth chart, but I recommend reading all the way through. You
may want to flip directly to your own Sun or rising sign (or a lover's if
·you're seeking to better understand them or help them achieve a healthier
sexuality). This is a perfectly fine way to use this book! But *Sex and Your
Stars* is best read from beginning to end, or at least picked up anew each
time we enter a new astrological season (I'm referring to the colloquially
used "Aries season," "Taurus season," etc.). Aries season, as I mentioned
in the introduction, begins on the vernal equinox around March 21, and
the remaining eleven signs' seasons follow until we come back around to
Aries again, as the Earth orbits the Sun every twelve months. That's what
we're really talking about with those ubiquitous memes and social media
hashtags referring to the season or *szn*.

Unlike many astrology books, *Sex and Your Stars* is experiential. In addition to reading (and potentially rereading) your own signs' chapters and

practicing the exercises there, you may want to take this book on a journey through the astrological seasons, digging into the energy of the moment, whenever and wherever you are when you find this book in your hands. The sign-by-sign chapters are designed to enhance and open your erotic journey through the year, as solar energies shift and change, and our minds and bodies respond. This might also be a fun and enlightening partner activity!

So, for example, when Cancer season begins on June 21 at the summer solstice, you can read the Cancer chapter, use the journaling questions and do the exercise(s), no matter what sign you are or the makeup of your natal chart. I also recommend reading the section on erogenous zones seasonally, as you may find that certain areas of your body are lit up when the Sun is moving through a corresponding sign. Even if you're an Aquarius or a Scorpio, the energy of the current season may feel compelling and relevant and offer you a sexual reset. When working with the seasons, pay attention to the erotic gifts section of the corresponding sign, as these are the energies you can tap into as the we journey around the Sun. Whatever your own Sun sign or rising sign, you can use this book to connect to the erotic energy of the moment, making it accessible to you as the astrological seasons change.

*Sex and Your Stars* can be understood as less literal and more energetic, based on the ancient tenets of Western astrology and its adherence to seasonal shifts as they were when this kind of astrology first developed. The references I reach for—from mentions of "sweater weather" in November to going for ice cream in July—are grounded in my experience growing up in the Northeastern United States. Yours may be different, but the astrological seasons can still elicit the same feelings, longings, and erotic shifts in all of us. To that end, though, we must acknowledge that the seasons as we've known them are not the same as they once were. Because our planet is quickly and dangerously warming, the April of now is not the April of most of our childhoods. The detailed descriptions of the seasons in each chapter might not directly resonate with your experience—not just because of the disconcerting ways that Decembers in New York City now have several 70-degree days, for example, but because you grew up in South Florida, and never had a cold winter. But even if I'm talking about a season of ice and snow that you might have only known as one where you drank iced tea on the porch, you should still be able to vibe with the overall energy of the description.

## Working and Playing Your Way Through This Book

Each of the twelve zodiac sign chapters of *Sex and Your Stars* is divided into eight sections. The first section covers the basics: the dates, sexual archetype, motivation, symbol, planetary ruler, element, modality, and the erogenous zone and body rulership of each sign. (More on what some of these terms mean below.) The second offers a general overview of the sign and its main attributes, with the third section offering an exploration of the sign's season and planetary ruler.

The fourth section dives into the erotic gifts of each sign. Because there is a deep, abiding, and fundamental relationship between the erotic and creative impulse in our body-minds as well as in many an astrologer's theory and practice, I briefly explore each sign's relationship with creativity in the "Pathway to Play" sections. The fifth section covers erotic challenges. The sixth delves into shame and shadow work to address those challenges and journaling questions to explore them. Both the erotic challenges and shame and shadow work sections include client stories. (Please note: all client names and identifying details in this book have been changed.) The seventh section covers the sign's body rulership and erogenous zones and how to elicit the most pleasure by focusing on them. The final section of the sign chapters offers embodiment exercises, rituals, or meditations tailored to each sign and season. Remember: you can pick up this book and flip to a specific sign to learn more about the planetary placements in your own or a lover's chart, AND you can read it as the astrological seasons shift, diving deep into the energy offered by each sign as you live within and experience it, learning more about your desires in the process.

After we move through the signs, we explore the pleasures of Venus, Mars, and Black Moon Lilith. The conclusion deepens our understanding of communication in sexual relationships and astrological counseling, and its fundamental role in sexual sovereignty, health, and pleasure, and gives a look ahead at the cosmic generational shifts of the next few decades—and how it might affect our erotic experiences.

The embodiment practices in this book draw on a range of tools and traditions, including clinical sexology, somatic experiencing, and yoga. I offer these as a way to help you regulate your nervous system and feel safe in your body—essential for grounding yourself in erotic experiences. I refer to these practices as exercises, but some of them may feel like sacred rituals to you, as I also drew from my own spiritual well of witchcraft, a practice I began exploring in my early twenties. I want to make clear that there is always danger of trafficking in cultural appropriation when we plumb concepts and language that are not from our own cultural traditions. However, I reference certain concepts like *chakras* (a term to describe the energetic pathways of the body that originated in India and comes from the Sanskrit word "wheel") or suggest some simple yoga poses in certain chapters in order to provide a way to physically access the embodiment exercises. The chakra system originated between 1500 and 500 BCE in a Hindu text called the Vedas. The second or sacral chakra is thought to be connected to our sexuality and desire, so it's integral to a number of the embodiment exercises I've created. This description of the sacral chakra and pleasure from Serina Payan Hazelwood comes from the chapter, "Yoga, A Liberatory Praxis" in one of the most important new books of the sexology pantheon, *The People's Book of Human Sexuality: Expanding the Sexology Archive*, edited by Bianca I. Laureano. (I urge all sexuality professionals to read this seminal text.)

> Like a bowl, the womb carries the memories of our ances-
> tors. Memories include trauma, pain, joy, and pleasure.
> These memories are important because they connect us to
> the roots that support our bodies and spirit in the ecosys-
> tem of life. Ancient yoga philosophy refers to the womb
> as Svadhisthana (sweetness), the sacral chakra. The sacral
> chakra represents sexuality, movement, life force, creation,
> restoration, and pleasure. Pleasure is our birthright and
> pathway to liberation. When humans embody pleasure,
> we are free and in our power.

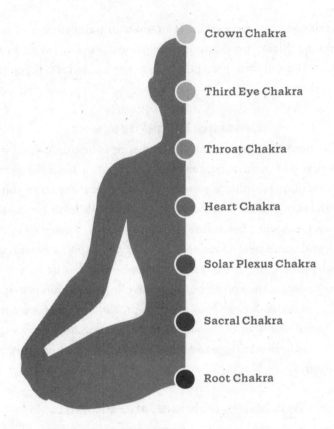

Crown Chakra

Third Eye Chakra

Throat Chakra

Heart Chakra

Solar Plexus Chakra

Sacral Chakra

Root Chakra

If you want to learn more about the history of the chakra system, you may want to read *Chakras: Energy Centers for Transformation*, by the late Indian scholar Harish Johari.

I've been a student of yoga for several decades, but I'm still a white person (with Ashkenazi Jewish roots from all over Europe) and I take note of my privilege here. Yoga is an Indian tradition that goes back more than five thousand years and is far more than just a fitness regime, but an entire way of life. The Indian continent was violently colonized by the British, and we must acknowledge that their culture is a *living culture* and it's not ours, as people of other cultures, to play with. As Westerners, it's essential to honor these traditions without defaulting to cultural misappropriation. I do my best with that in these pages, always keeping in mind that there is an uncomfortable history of white people taking Black, brown, and indigenous people's ideas, history, and culture and not only pretending that they created it but profiting off that creation.

## Creating Ritual Space

Since this book is experiential, most chapters include embodiment exercises that, as I mentioned, may feel like rituals. I've aimed to make these as easy and accessible as possible and have set them up so you can work with them exactly where you are. This book is about sexuality, and the exercises will often call for privacy—ideally, a space you can go to and spend some time alone to deepen your relationship with your body and your chart. This is also a privilege—some of us have young kids, work long hours (often both), or live in small, cramped spaces with other humans. So again, as much as possible, if you have a room in your home where you can have privacy, or time to use a common room when others aren't around, that will help you to use this book experientially.

## Disability, Ableism, and Pleasure

I will say it again and again: all humans deserve pleasure. Disability itself is not a problem: it's an identity and a culture, and disabled people continue to fight to be seen. Ableism is so deeply embedded in our language that we often barely know it's there. The exercises and embodiment practices in this book may call for movement and sensory awareness that may not be available to all people, but I invite readers to interpret and use them wherever they are right now, in whatever ways feel comfortable and safe as they journey toward understanding their sexual selves. The resources section includes accessibility-minded sexual enhancement tools.

You might also notice that rather than addressing the reader as "you" in the sign and planet chapters, I make space for however you might find yourself coming to this book. So in the Scorpio chapter, for instance, I might say "Scorpios may enjoy . . ." or "The Scorpio tends to feel . . ."

or "Scorpio people often experience . . ." or "Scorpio erotic energy gives off . . ." depending on the context. The point, in part, is that none of this is prescribed—it's all about the energy of potentials, endlessly fluid and malleable.

We may feel much like our sign during one particular year of our lives and lean more deeply into another part of our chart at a different stage (depending on transits and life experiences). Remember that in this book I'm offering an aspirational analysis that tunes into the essential *erotic vitality* of each sign. Trusting your own experience above all is the key, both in the realm of astrology and sexology. If a sentence or paragraph doesn't resonate with you, there is nothing wrong with you. This might just be a sign from the universe that you should go deeper into your own chart and explore the source of your erotic energy or challenges.

## Understanding Signs, Seasons, and Elements

As we move through the twelve signs, exploring the intimate psychological nuances of each astrological archetype, you may notice that I refer to the previous sign's season and traits, and refer to other signs that share the same *element* or *modality*. In the way that I work with the tropical zodiac, each sign tends to course correct for the excesses of the previous sign, as if they're in an ongoing conversation. We can learn a lot about how it feels to live in a hot and active Aries body when we begin to study the other fire signs or the other cardinal signs, and we may learn a lot about what it means to be a more controlled Capricorn when we look at the excesses of their predecessor Sagittarius, and so forth.

Let's explore how I break down the energetic assignations of the signs in the simplest way, but with a bit more detail to support you as you journey through the astrological seasons. Our zodiac's seasons begin with Aries around March 21—the astrological New Year and the start of spring in the Northern Hemisphere, opening with the vernal or spring equinox, and lasting approximately thirty days. In tropical astrology, each sign is associated with one of four natural elements—fire, earth, air, or water.

The fire signs are Aries, Leo, and Sagittarius.

The earth signs are Taurus, Virgo, and Capricorn.

The air signs are Gemini, Libra, and Aquarius.

The water signs are Cancer, Scorpio, and Pisces.

Each sign also has a *modality*, which describes the way the sign interacts or moves within the world.

The *cardinal* signs are Aries, Cancer, Libra, and Capricorn. These signs create, spark, and initiate.

The *fixed* signs are Taurus, Leo, Scorpio, and Aquarius. These signs deepen, hold, and preserve.

The *mutable* signs are Gemini, Virgo, Sagittarius, and Pisces. These signs integrate, move dynamically, flow, and transform.

Sometimes it helps to visualize the elements and their modes, to get a better, more embodied sense of the way they work together.

## Visualizing the Elements

| Fire Signs | Earth Signs | Air Signs | Water Signs |
|---|---|---|---|
| **Aries** (cardinal): a match striking | **Taurus** (fixed): a spring meadow in bloom | **Gemini** (mutable): a synapse firing | **Cancer** (cardinal): waves ebbing and flowing on the shore |
| **Leo** (fixed): a bonfire on the beach | **Virgo** (mutable): a perfectly tilled garden of fresh healing herbs | **Libra** (cardinal): a one-on-one conversation | **Scorpio** (fixed): a cauldron simmering to a boil |
| **Sagittarius** (mutable): an uncontrolled wildfire | **Capricorn** (cardinal): a rocky mountain face with a path to the peak | **Aquarius** (fixed): an idea that moves humanity forward | **Pisces** (mutable): an entire ocean |

## Houses and House Systems

If you're new to astrology, you may not be familiar with the word *house* as it's used in this field, and even though I don't deal directly with house placements in this book, it's worth briefly touching on what they are and how they work. As discussed earlier, the time of your birth determines the exact degree of the sign on the eastern horizon of your chart, known as the ascendant or rising sign. If the signs tell you *who* you are, the houses tell you *the area of life* in which you are the way you are. If you have planets in a particular house, their energetic purpose remains the same—for example, Venus may have an association with love, romance, and pleasure. The sign it's in will tell us how that Venus *feels*. A Venus in Pisces might tend to fall in love with love and experience romance as a kind of ethereal poetry, and also be willing to make huge sacrifices for their lover(s). But if we also know that Venus is in the eleventh house, ruling our social relationships, that Venus in Pisces might exist in a person who falls in love with their friends, for example. Every sign has thirty degrees, and depending on the house system an astrologer is using, the houses may be intercepted by more than one sign.

In sexual and relationship astrology, all houses are relevant, because our sexuality is threaded through our entire existence. But the fifth house (the house of pleasure and play, or as I sometimes refer to it, "The Tinder House"), the seventh house (the partnership and marriage house, ruling contracts and one-to-one relationships), and the eighth house (ruling deep, transformative experiences, subversive sexual experiences, and sometimes, sexual trauma) are often linked to our sexuality and erotic experiences across our lifetimes. There is a lot of controversy around the eighth house! Many astrologers will say it has nothing to do with sex because it's a house of loss, but my perspective, again, is that ALL houses relate to our sexuality in some way, because we can't compartmentalize sexuality into a limited realm of our lives. Our sexuality is always a part of us, even when we're at work (the domain of the sixth house) or talking on the phone (the domain of the third house). In my experience, transits to the fifth, seventh, and eighth houses can fundamentally shift our perspective on our sexuality and our sex lives.

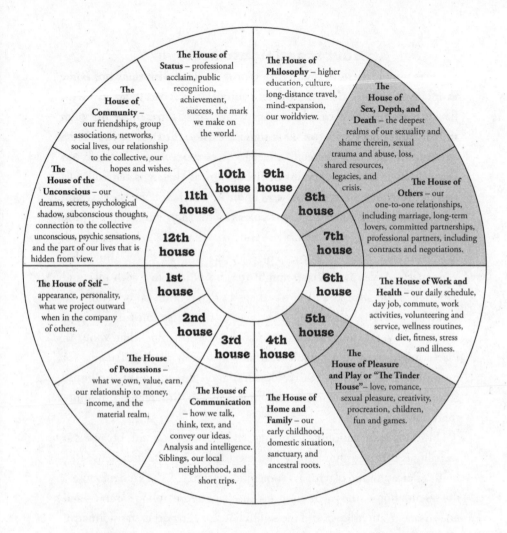

The House of Status – professional acclaim, public recognition, achievement, success, the mark we make on the world.

The House of Community – our friendships, group associations, networks, social lives, our relationship to the collective, our hopes and wishes.

The House of Philosophy – higher education, culture, long-distance travel, mind-expansion, our worldview.

The House of Sex, Depth, and Death – the deepest realms of our sexuality and shame therein, sexual trauma and abuse, loss, shared resources, legacies, and crisis.

The House of the Unconscious – our dreams, secrets, psychological shadow, subconscious thoughts, connection to the collective unconscious, psychic sensations, and the part of our lives that is hidden from view.

The House of Others – our one-to-one relationships, including marriage, long-term lovers, committed partnerships, professional partners, including contracts and negotiations.

The House of Self – appearance, personality, what we project outward when in the company of others.

The House of Work and Health – our daily schedule, day job, commute, work activities, volunteering and service, wellness routines, diet, fitness, stress and illness.

The House of Possessions – what we own, value, earn, our relationship to money, income, and the material realm.

The House of Communication – how we talk, think, text, and convey our ideas. Analysis and intelligence. Siblings, our local neighborhood, and short trips.

The House of Home and Family – our early childhood, domestic situation, sanctuary, and ancestral roots.

The House of Pleasure and Play or "The Tinder House"– love, romance, sexual pleasure, creativity, procreation, children, fun and games.

10th house
9th house
11th house
8th house
12th house
7th house
1st house
6th house
2nd house
5th house
3rd house
4th house

It gets a lot more complicated, but to put it simply for our purposes in this book, different astrologers use a variety of house systems with all different kinds of mathematical calculations to determine what a chart looks like and where planets and points fall. I generally use Placidus and Whole Sign systems when I cast charts. If you go to a site like astro.com or use an app to find out what your rising sign is, or where any of the planets live in your chart, you might want to check to see what house system is being used. Astro.com will allow you to adjust it to your preference.

## Essential Dignities

You'll notice that when I describe the planets in signs, I may use words like **domicile**, **detriment**, **exaltation**, and **fall**. This is a traditional astrology concept, also used by modern astrologers, that tells us more about the health of the planets depending on what sign they are in. I'm super-simplifying the concept here, but domicile is a planet's comfort zone, exaltation is a planet's happy place, where it can live up to its highest potential, detriment is where a planet feels uncomfortable, and fall is where a planet's hardest challenges can become its successes with hard work.

| Essential Dignities Simplified, Including Traditional and Modern Rulership | | | | |
|---|---|---|---|---|
| Sign | Domicile + | Exaltation + | Detriment - | Fall - |
| Aries | Mars | Sun | Venus | Saturn |
| Taurus | Venus | Moon | Mars | None |
| Gemini | Mercury | None | Jupiter | None |
| Cancer | Moon | Jupiter | Saturn | Mars |
| Leo | Sun | None | Saturn | None |
| Virgo | Mercury | Mercury | Jupiter | Venus |
| Libra | Venus | Saturn | Mars | Sun |
| Scorpio | Mars/Pluto | None | Venus | Moon |
| Sagittarius | Jupiter | None | Mercury | None |
| Capricorn | Saturn | Mars | Moon | Jupiter |
| Aquarius | Saturn/Uranus | None | Sun | None |
| Pisces | Jupiter/Neptune | Venus | Mercury | Mercury |

## Erogenous Zones and Body Rulerships

We have multiple erogenous zones beyond the genitals. Some people know their erogenous zones quite well, while others need to experiment to find them. Still others discover new ones across their lifetime or with new partners. Many people think of erogenous zones in terms of seduction, but this is the kind of discovery we can make on our own and later bring into partnered sex if we want to. You don't have to wait for anyone to show you—you can find your own body's secret pleasure spots, and astrology has much to tell us about how to stimulate them.

One of the many limitations our broader culture (and mainstream porn culture) forces on our relationship with our sexual selves is the idea that pleasure can only be experienced through the genitals, breasts, and perhaps the mouth. This gets a big old NOPE from me. Our erogenous zones are unlimited, and part of the fun of being alive and in a body is experimenting and discovering where they are and how to give them pleasure.

Astrology identifies sensitive or important parts of our body and its systems—what we refer to as *body rulership* by the associated sign. There is also a branch of astrology called medical astrology that is dedicated to the body and our health. There are endlessly complex medical delineations for each sign, planet, and aspect in a natal chart, plus all kinds of fascinating remedies for ailments, but my aim here is to simplify this concept while simultaneously broadening it to better represent the ways our bodies feel pleasure. In my work, when a client learns the body rulerships associated with their chart and begins to think of them as a source of potential pleasure, their relationship to their body shifts in a beautiful, positive way.

For example, Gemini rules the shoulders, arms, and hands. In medical astrology, this might be understood to suggest that Gemini natives are sensitive in these parts of their body, or perhaps that these appendages are prone to problems. In my experience, Geminis can feel pleasure in these areas and also provide pleasure for their lovers through them. We'll look more deeply at how sign-body rulership intersects with our erogenous zones in each sign-based chapter.

## Pause and Breathe with Me

A note about breathing—in life, sex, and for the exercises in this book. Breathing is something we're doing every minute we're alive, as it's a function controlled by our autonomic or involuntary nervous system. But our breath is often shallow and disordered and not serving the rest of our bodies well. Becoming aware of the breath can change so much about your experience of your body, your emotional tenor, your sense of safety, and your relationship to pleasure.

However, often when we're instructed to breathe a certain way, as in a yoga class or in exercises that call for deeper breaths into certain regions of the body, we can become anxious about doing it right, which makes it harder for us to relax and actually connect to our breath. It's a vicious cycle and it takes practice to become aware of the breath without worrying. I invite you into softness and gentleness when it comes to your relationship with your breath, rather than getting overly caught up in the instructions about breathing in the exercises in this book. If any of them feel too detailed or take you out of your body, just relax and breathe normally.

One of the reasons I never do prerecorded readings is because the energetic flow between me and my client is essential, and our bodies are the conduit in somatic work. Breathing is an essential part of this process. Even if we're on Zoom or a call, I want to be able to tune into a client's nervous system and help them get grounded. And I allow all of my Aries fire to come through, so the client can feel my enthusiasm about their process and know that I know they can heal. I hope that as you read this book, you'll feel my earnest excitement about the future of your sex life, and how much pleasure is ahead for you. Think of me as your cheerleader, swinging around red pompoms and sparklers.

## On Trauma and Sexual Trauma

We live in an age of relentless trauma, and my work is trauma-informed. Humans, of course, have never escaped trauma, and the fight-or-flight mechanism built into our nervous system is thought to have evolved because of the physical dangers early humans were exposed to on an everyday basis. Despite the truly remarkable expansion of our lifespans thanks to the technologies of modern medicine, indoor plumbing, etc., we have grown more anxious and depressed in the twenty-first century. White supremacy, fascism, capitalism, climate change, constant exposure to screens screeching scary headlines—so many sources contribute to the trauma we carry in our bodies. This trauma separates us from the sensations that can connect us to our erotic gifts.

For those who have experienced sexual trauma, this stress is compounded. An analysis of prevalence data from 2001–2018 across 161 countries conducted by the World Health Organization (WHO) showed that 30 percent of women aged 15–49—that's one in three—had experienced sexual abuse or intimate partner violence.[1] Sexual trauma can make it even harder to navigate relationships and sex—including the sex we have with ourselves. This is to say that you may come to this book with more complex trauma issues to unpack, and I hope that you're getting or intend to get the kind of support you need to navigate your path to pleasure. I highly recommend a wonderful book called *With Pleasure: Managing Trauma Triggers for More Vibrant Sex and Relationships* by August McLaughlin and Jamila Dawson, LMFT.

## Let's Talk About Sex! (and Pleasure)

Sex education is scant in most societies and increasingly so in the United States, where frighteningly retrograde ideas about sexuality are on the rise in many states and being codified into law by state legislatures. As theocratic governments across the world force their citizens to live under fundamentalist conditions (and others grope toward authoritarianism), sexual pleasure is one of the first rights we lose.

This is a grave shame, as according to the WHO, sexual pleasure is a human right. The desire for intimacy with ourselves and others is a fundamental human need. This is another way of saying that sexual pleasure is a PART OF GOOD HEALTH, and good health is a human right. There should be nothing controversial about this. We tend to think of sexual pleasure as something separate and apart from "health," even sexual health (avoiding sexually transmitted infections (STIs), understanding birth control, etc.). But few people think of getting a green smoothie or going for their annual physical the same way they think of having an orgasm.

I cannot begin to tell you the number of times I've said, "an orgasm a day keeps the doctor away"—because if I'm a fundamentalist about anything, it's the ways in which pleasure can heal us both in body and mind. Pleasure is a word I'll come back to again and again in this book—it's perhaps the most important word of all, and it is something we all deserve.

Let's define some other terms that you'll see in these pages, ones that I use every day in my practice.

**Consent:** Consent is sexual permission, i.e., when all people involved in a sexual activity agree to choose to take part. Consent is usually given by word or action. Affirmative or *enthusiastic consent* adds a layer of YES! to consent, showing that you're excited about the activity that you're about to participate in. One important factor about consent: all parties must understand that it can be withdrawn at any time.

**Erotic:** The Greek word *eros* means "physical love or sexual desire." Simply defined, *erotic* means "arousing sexual feelings or desires." In her essential essay "The Uses of the Erotic: The Erotic as Power," Audre Lorde says, "The erotic is a measure between the beginnings of our sense of self and the chaos of our strongest feelings. It is an internal sense of satisfaction to which, once we have experienced it, we know we can aspire. For having experienced the fullness of this depth of feeling and recognizing its power, in honor and self-respect we can require no less of ourselves."

Passion, love, lust, and romance all fall under its umbrella. Some call this "limerence" or new relationship energy. According to Freud, Eros is the life instinct innate in all humans, and the opposite of Thanatos, the death drive. When I write about erotic gifts and challenges in this book, it's partly with these concepts in mind.

**Libido:** This is the Latin word for desire, and it's been through a number of iterations since the field of sexology first emerged a little more than a century ago. It's sometimes used interchangeably with eros, as well. I prefer *libido* or *sexual motivation* to *sex drive*, because the latter can be loaded and misused. If you prefer or are used to the term *sex drive*, that's fine! The most important thing to understand about libido is that it fluctuates from human to human and across one's lifetime. You may think yours is problematic, but it's more than likely just fine, and this book can help you reignite yours if it's been waning.

**Shadow and Shadow Work:** This is a concept derived from the psychoanalytic work of Carl Jung, where our shadow is the hidden, unconscious, denied part of our psyche that we often must work hard to recognize and honor. In astrology, a simple shorthand exists for our shadow—we can look at the traits of the opposite sign to reveal it.

**Toxic Masculinity:** A patriarchal culture that glorifies male dominance and, often, violence and is harmful to all people.

**Asexuality:** Some people do not experience sexual feelings and desires (and this does not mean they are broken). Asexuals or "aces" often still experience feelings of love and long for romantic attachments and partnerships. This book is primarily designed for those who do experience sexual desire and want to better understand its complexities, but I've included some tools for those who identify as asexual in the resources section.

**Cis or Cisgender:** A person who identifies with their gender assignment at birth. When I refer to someone who is both cisgender and heterosexual, I often use the informal term *cishet*.

**Trans:** A person who does not solely identify with both the sex they were assigned at birth and the gender socially associated with that sex.

**Ethical Non-Monogamy or ENM:** Ethical non-monogamy (sometimes referred to as consensual non-monogamy or CNM) is the umbrella term used for the practice of being romantically or sexually involved with multiple people *who all agree with this relationship structure*. Even though these relationships are increasingly common, there is still a lot of stigma around them. In ENM relationships, there is a core commitment to communication, consideration, and consent.

**Open Relationships:** Open relationships are generally when monogamous partners open up their relationship to dating or having sex with other partners.

**Polyamory:** The primary focus of polyamorous relationships is love or romantic feelings between multiple partners, but not necessarily sex (although sex is often a part of these relationships). Some people consider polyamory to be an orientation, not just an intimate practice or identity, akin to a sexual orientation.

**Kink/BDSM:** Kink is any kind of nonconventional sexual practice. BDSM kink practices often involve a consensual exchange of power.

*Normal* is a word that has been used in harmful ways, so I want to be clear what I mean when I use it here. It suggests that anything outside of society's bounds should be pathologized, yet sometimes the word *normal* can be helpful and even necessary in certain contexts. The concept of *normalcy* is firmly baked into the way we see and interact with the world, and although we may eventually edit it out of our vocabulary when it comes to sexuality, that hasn't happened yet.

We might tease apart our relationship to what is "normal" for us by interrogating the parts of our desire that were formed before we had a deeper understanding of patriarchal dynamics, for instance. Patriarchy, to me, is far from normal, but it is the paradigm in which we all live, even as we're fighting to deconstruct and dismantle it. Even when there are tension, confusion, and the sense that your sexual feelings contradict your social justice values, there should be no shame.

Speaking of the vagaries of what is "normal," I want to make space for how normal it is for people of ALL AGES, including people over forty, in perimenopause, post-menopausal, and yes, senior citizens, to feel desire and have sex—sometimes quite a bit of it! We are sexual beings from birth to death, and even as our bodies change and slow down, that remains. We desperately need to reduce shame around our bodies as we age, and, more specifically for this book, the way that aging bodies experience themselves erotically. You'll notice that several of the client stories I include in this book are about people that society might consider "old" or "mature." They are in this book for a good reason, because their sex lives and access to pleasure matter.

When I discuss what other clinicians might call *sexual dysfunction*, I prefer to use the terms *sexual concern* or *sexual issue*. You can start to see how shame emerges just in the language we've traditionally used to frame our sexuality, and why terms that seem simple and innocuous can be problematic. Whether it's low libido, anorgasmia (common for vulva-havers), erectile concerns for penis-havers (including premature and delayed erection or difficulty experiencing erection), mismatched desire (in partnerships), desire for enhanced pleasure, social inhibitions, or dating deficits, all the concerns I see in my practice are widely shared, but each client tends to feel isolated, as if they're the only person in the world experiencing their issue. There are tons more, and while every situation is unique, the most common, universal theme is that my clients are carrying a lot of shame.

*Healthy* is also a complicated word in our society, sometimes conferring a moral implication, and one that I strongly disagree with. Yet when used as an adjective to describe signs or planets in astrology, it can be effective and meaningful—I'll often use it to reference an individual sign's energetic potentials. In this context, *healthy* means unblocked, unobstructed, robust, clear, and uninhibited: strong in the natal chart. In any chart, a planet's inherent power can be minimized by hard aspects, house placement, challenging transits, and other more complex astrological phenomena. So, in using the word *healthy*, I'm referring to the higher potential of a sign or planetary placement—not necessarily what it feels like to live with that astrological signature every day.

## Smashing Shame, Season by Season

Guilt is just as powerful, but its influence is positive, while shame's is destructive. Shame erodes our courage and fuels disengagement.

**Brené Brown**

"Listening to Shame"

My work around sex and sexual health is rooted in the concept of holistic or *embodied sexuality*, a broad term that, for me, describes moving toward a sexuality that is focused on pleasure, sensuality, and whole-body awareness. My version of embodied sexuality requires an interrogation of shame, guilt, and self-judgment. I actively reject the harmful heteropatriarchal mores that keep us bound in ideas about how we should look and feel and tell us that only certain kinds of sex and desire are sanctioned. When we witness and practice this through the lens of astrological seasons, we can begin to appreciate all the complicated, delicious layers of our erotic selves.

As you work through the book seasonally, you may find that some exercises bring out a sign's natural energy while others rely on the sign's polarity. For instance, the exercises for the fire signs (Aries, Leo, and Sagittarius) may be more activating and erotically energizing, but the air sign exercises (Gemini, Libra, and Aquarius) aren't necessarily intellectual and heady, like their signs' natures. Rather, some exercises are designed to bring our focus out of our heads and back to the physical or emotional body. In other words, not every sign-season exercise brings out *more* of the energy of that sign. This is because in sexual embodiment work, I aim to take you deeper into your body and help you to get out of your head and the kind of analysis paralysis that can block pleasure.

Often our very first erotic impulses, what turned us on before we could make any sense of it, before we could identify it as toxic or dangerous or shameful, is what continues to create a kind of libidinous frisson into adulthood. Our sexual history is nothing to be ashamed of or to strip out or destroy. In my experience, we tend to add additional layers to our desire matrix before we erase the old. And often, we never fully erase those earlier layers, even the problematic ones, but instead find ways to heal and integrate them.

When I use the word *sex* in this book as a verb, as in "to have sex," I am not just talking about intercourse. Sex can be kissing, foreplay, oral/anal pleasure, use of sex toys, penetration with fingers and other objects, arousal in or with nature (such as the emerging discipline of ecosex/ecosexuality), etc. There is a persistent and annoying assumption that *sex* means intercourse, or what we sexologists refer to as P-in-V (penis in vagina) sex. Penis-in-vagina sex is a great kind of sex! I'm not knocking it. I'm just saying that sex is whatever you want to do, solo or with a partner, with whatever bodies or body parts that turn you on and make you feel good and give your body pleasure.

Speaking of pleasure, or what some consider the ultimate pleasure of sex—let's talk briefly about orgasms. I want to make it clear that although orgasms are GREAT and I want you to have a lot of them if you want them, they too are not the be-all-end-all of sex. Some people are content to cuddle, fondle, kiss, and massage a partner and skip the orgasm, or touch themselves in all kinds of pleasurable ways without coming. (Note: I do not use the word *cum* as a verb—for me, cum is the substance of ejaculatory fluid, and yes, I realize this is nonstandard.) Some people like to fool around with a partner many times before they provide or experience an orgasm, building up that tension. And some people like to have orgasms every day—even more than once, both by themselves and with lovers! You might be anywhere on that spectrum, and this is totally okay.

## What Exactly Is an Orgasm?

The first thing to understand about orgasms is that they happen in the brain, not the genitals. Sex researchers and scientists still don't have a conclusive, agreed-upon definition of what's happening biologically at the moment of orgasm, but I prefer the simple definition of an orgasm from Emily Nagoski, author of the seminal book *Come As You Are* (a text I'll mention more than once in *Sex and Your Stars*): "Orgasm is the spontaneous, involuntary release of tension generated in response to sex-related stimuli."

The nuances of the sexual response cycle are covered beautifully in books like Nagoski's and others I'll include in the resources section, but what I want you to know now is that orgasms are spectacularly diverse. Like sexuality itself, they exist on a spectrum, with some orgasms feeling like a soft but pleasant sneeze and some feeling like an earthquake of vibrating pleasure that can be a bit overwhelming. Please never feel shame about the kind of orgasms you have, have had, or hope to have. They tend to change across one's lifetime and can improve as we regulate our nervous system and address mental and emotional blocks. Remember, orgasm happens in the brain, and our brains can be trained.

The essential path to orgasm goes something like this: blood flows to the brain, the genital sensory cortex is activated, the brain's reward system lights up (cue the dopamine, serotonin, and oxytocin—the "happy hormones"), pain is inhibited, and then we plateau and may be ready to go again once we've rested up. One of the reasons I advocate for orgasms—lots of them, as often as possible—is because they're really good for our physical, mental, and emotional health. If you want to learn more about the science of orgasms and a lot of other juicy and meaningful information about sex, I encourage you to read Dr. Nan Wise's book *Why Good Sex Matters*.

Many of the exercises in this book make space for and encourage orgasm, and you might find that your relationship to your orgasmic potential may shift or strengthen, especially if you practice them regularly or use the book through the astrological seasons.

## The Issues I See in My Practice

The most common sexual concerns I see in my practice are desire issues, where someone has a lack of desire or interest in sex and sexual activities; arousal issues, where a client can't become physically excited, even if they want to have sex; orgasm issues, where someone experiences a delay or absence of orgasm; and pain issues, which I sometimes have to refer to another practitioner.

Our pain is complex and nuanced. Sometimes I can work through pain concerns with a client through therapeutic reflection and somatic exercises, and sometimes pain concerns need additional kinds of support from medical doctors like urologists or gynecologists, pelvic support specialists like pelvic floor therapists, trauma therapists like EMDR practitioners, or massage therapists, acupuncturists, and naturopaths. I want to validate that your pain concerns are real and important! I hope this book offers meaningful support, and I also encourage you to reach out for personal or medical care when needed. I offer resources at the end of the book that might point you in a helpful direction.

It's important to understand that anyone of any sign, with any chart, can at some point in their lifetime experience *any type of sexual issue*. Please don't read these chapters and assume you have a predilection for say, delayed ejaculation or low desire because the story in the chapter that matches your sign is about a client with those challenges. The shame and trauma we experience in our family dynamic, culture, and relationships are not chart dependent, but our astrological makeup can help us navigate *how we meet and deal with that shame*.

When I assess a sex coaching client, I use my mentor Dr. Patti Britton's remarkable, holistic, efficient MEBES™ model, in which I evaluate their mind or mental state (M), their emotions (E), their behaviors/body (B), their energy (E), and their spirit/spirituality (S). Then I define the breakdown and create an action plan for the client. Although I'm not formally meeting with the readers of this book, I want the chapters to serve as templates for you to observe your own mind/body/emotions/spirit in whatever sequence feels right for you. Whether you're having a sexual issue or are just here to understand yourself better as a sexual being and experience more pleasure through the seasons of the astrological year and your life, these pages can serve as a guide.

We deepen and grow into our sexual selves by paying attention to our desire, by listening to it, and by responding to it instead of shutting it down, not by judging or fearing parts of it. This book invites us to engage with it all, even the parts we'd rather hide from, so we can draw out the power and pleasure of our erotic gifts.

Something I think and talk about a lot (possibly because my Sun is in Aries—more on this in the next chapter) is that all humans are mammals, which is to say—we are animals. And one thing we know about animals is that when they feel safe, they often play. I invite you to remember that you, too, are an animal, and to seek the kind of safety and security that will allow your sex life to become a place of play.

This book's purpose is to help you become sexually embodied and fulfilled, using the astrological archetypes as guides. *Sex and Your Stars* can help you identify your desires and work with your challenges to deepen your connection to yourself and to others. The proverb at the beginning of the introduction, "As above, so below," speaks to me not just of the planets and the human lives they influence, but of the brain and the body. I hope this book both answers your burning questions and opens the doors of your perception, so you can choose to have even more pleasure.

# 2

# Aries Sexuality

## Energy and Exhilaration

At once a gentle fire has caught throughout my flesh, and
I see nothing with my eyes, and there's a drumming
in my ears, and sweat pours down on me . . .

**Sappho**

**Dates:** March 21–April 20

**Sexual Archetype:** The Hunter

**Motivation:** Lust

**Symbol:** The Ram

**Planetary Ruler:** Mars (also rules Scorpio)

**Element:** Fire

**Modality:** Cardinal

**Erogenous Zones and Body Rulership:** The Eyes,
Head, Face, Blood, and Adrenal Glands

Healthy Aries energy is fevered, passionate, courageous, insistent, untamed, eager, wildly confident, and fervently feral. Aries people may express their desires as a demand. As essential forces of nature, they love to assertively flirt. At their core, they've got BFE: big fire energy.

Yet when Aries are thwarted from pursuing their essential mission—living by their fierce instincts—their sexuality can become flat, frustrated, and exhausted. To keep their eternal flame lit, they must follow the fire of their intuition. Competition is the kinetic force that captures the erotic attention of an Aries, even when they're only competing against themselves.

## It's a Question of Lust: Aries Season in Focus

Aries is the very first sign of the zodiac; it's the fire-starter that lights the match of the world with its extraordinary zeal. When the Sun is in Aries, it can seem like the entire world instantly turns on. This is the beginning of the astrological year and the turning of the wheel of time once again. Aries is a cardinal fire sign, so initiation is unavoidable now. Sweaters are peeling off in much of the Northern Hemisphere, green shoots are sprouting up from underneath the soil, animals are beginning to beckon and call each other to mate. We humans can tap into a "stirring in the loins" sensation during this time of year, and it's especially helpful for curing the winter blahs or bringing a feeling of aliveness back to our sex lives—and our solo sex lives, whether we're partnered or single.

Sometimes Aries season can feel like waking up fully alert from a deep slumber, as our circadian rhythms begin to readjust to the expansion of the light. Subtly longer days activate parts of our bodies that have been asleep for months, in hibernation, waiting to be enlivened once again. We might tune into our senses in a new way, noticing attractive people on our path that we may have missed in the colder months, when our instinct was simply to get home faster to our warm, safe space. Now the outside is becoming safe and warm again, and our hunting instinct is turning back on.

Lust is frowned upon in many cultures, but during Aries season, I invite you to explore the ways it can free you to engage with your environment like an animal might, with no self-criticism—only your body's inclinations. It doesn't mean you have to act on them—but suppressing them doesn't do you any favors.

No matter your Sun sign, Aries season is an excellent time to tap into the instinctive part of your sexual self and awaken your animal urges, reengaging with your body in a fierce, fiery way. You may not have any planets in Aries, but Aries does live *somewhere* in your chart, and when the Sun (which is exalted in Aries) is there, it activates a particular house and life arena, as outlined in the section on houses in chapter 2.

## Get to Know Mars, Aries' Planetary Ruler

If Mars had an ad slogan, it would probably be JUST MOVE. Mars is the planet of our will, our physicality, our passion, and sometimes, our rage. Mars energy is what gets us out of the house in the morning to go for a run. Mars is what drives us to speak up when someone is pissing us off. Mars is what gives us the courage to pursue a lover when we're not fully confident that they're interested in us. Mars is what it feels like when lust rises up in us like fire. Mars thrusts and must always move forward. When blocked or held back, this energy can shape itself into a dagger, one that might prick the people around us, or even ourselves. Mars also rules Scorpio, and chapter 15 is entirely dedicated to the Red Planet.

## Aries' Erotic Gifts

When fully expressed, Aries energy is the astrological embodiment of pure, unhindered libido. Aries lust can feel like a primal scream; Rams express the sound and fury of being born ready for anything. Their legendary impatience can be quite off-putting to the uninitiated, especially for more sensitive types. But when an Aries bursts into flames in pursuit of something they desire—that is erotic power in action. Even when Aries, arguably the most sexual of signs, is taking out the garbage, feeding the cat, or ordering a coffee, something about their action feels *primal*—sometimes to both the Aries native and anyone in their midst.

Certain Aries can seem to be suspended in a state of beginner's mind, as if they're trying everything for the first time—including sex and intimacy (solo or partnered). In fact, Aries humans sometimes seem to *need* this first-time-feeling to become aroused, both in fantasy and reality.

One of the erotic gifts unique to Aries people is their guilelessness when it comes to sex and pleasure. They're not usually capable of playing it cool when turned on. In love and lust, a healthy Aries' sexual philosophy is straightforward: why be anything less than fearless when there is only the moment in front of you? Even if a Ram is not a trained meditator, they sometimes seem like they've mastered the art of the Tao—they will not waste a single precious moment.

Rams may quickly size up potential paramours—they may not know they're quite literally sniffing people out, but as the Hunter archetype, Aries will often know whether they want someone as soon as they get close enough to smell them. Aries can be so bound to their physicality that pheromones will often do this work for them subconsciously; it's rarely an intellectual process. Even if they have no idea whether they'll get it right in the end, if they're in touch with their erotic gifts, Aries are often willing to try and fail when it comes to going after what their bodies want.

Aries often make snap decisions about love and sex based on the fire of instant intuition—and this is something we can tap into during Aries season. Why ponder or meander when you can just . . . go get it? When Aries people feel something, they're not great at waiting for circumstances to play out. This is why they often start new projects (and relationships) with zeal but give up rather quickly when it appears that additional work might be necessary. Aries are great with intention; follow-up, not so much. This isn't necessarily problematic unless they actively make promises but fail to keep them when they get bored or see other potential lovers on the path, so they can start the hunt all over again. Yet whether they're pushing for sexual or creative release, a healthy Aries is not likely to waste anyone's time.

To unlock Aries desire, the precept is simple: directness rules. All humans are mammals, but Aries humans tend to function more like animals than any other sign. They are primal beings, and, like the Rams who are their zodiacal symbol, they often thrill to the chase. They can be turned on in record speed, as soon as their skin is touched, or if they're told or shown that they're wanted—via text, carrier pigeon, or a morning erection. They can be impulsive, with desire often elicited in seconds. When operating on the responsive desire scale, a healthy Aries can turn on more quickly than other signs. *Responsive desire*, a term developed by Dr. Emily Nagoski, is desire that happens in reaction to sexual stimuli, after arousal, and is more common for vulva-owners than penis-owners. I explore this in more detail in the Mars chapter.

Aries is probably the sign most likely to want to keep masturbating even when they're having partnered sex often. They might bring themselves to orgasm next to their partner in bed if they haven't been properly gotten off before going to sleep. When they're feeling well and life is unburdened by other vexing issues, Aries are almost always ready to go, and to exhaust their partners anew. The erotic energy of a healthy Aries human can be depleted by trauma, grief, and eventually, by aging, but even then, not as much as you might expect. Yes, Aries septuagenarians often see no reason not to keep their sexual fires burning even as some of their age cohort go without.

Learning to unapologetically own and love their animal nature and recognizing, affirming, and continuously experiencing this instinctual fervor supports a satisfying sex life for Rams. And for Aries, more than any other sign, a good sex life translates into a good life.

## Pathway to Play and Creativity for Aries

Aries rules the head, and creative explosions tend to burst forward through their craniums like a fireworks display. There are so many ideas, happening so fast and loud, that it can be difficult to keep track of them. This is before they've even laid down a foundation, and certainly before any focusing and finishing has taken place. I recommend that Aries keep a notebook with them at all times, have their phone's recording app at the ready, or text themselves any little snippets of ideas so they can eventually make some sense of them. The key to Aries creativity is not just initially touching that fire of intuition, but finding a way to sustain it for the long(er) haul. They must learn to be patient with themselves when too many ideas come at once and crowd each other out. Mind-mapping and other creative organizational principles might be useful.

Even something as simple as using brightly colored Post-its in their work area can help order their blazing brains. Aries' creative instincts can thrive with artistic mediums that require some physicality—like Jackson Pollock–style drip painting, sculpting, and dancing. But they might use these just as a jumping off point for some other creative endeavor.

## Aries' Erotic Challenges

In order for an Aries to be in their sexual element and tap the confidence within them, they must first work through any shame they have experienced from restrictive or religious cultures. Whether we personally identify as religious or not, even the most secular, atheistic nonbelievers and those raised without religion can be steeped in this kind of shame, given how common this is across cultures. For Aries, a sign that doesn't really do the in-betweens, porn-or-purity messaging can create a major conundrum. Desire can feel threatening, because the first time they express it, the fiery enormity of it can cause blowback and shock from the people around them.

When we're born into a body that feels so intensely, overpoweringly, and fiercely libidinous as Aries bodies tend to be when at their most vital, it can be confusing when primal desires and instinctual responses are labeled taboo or "too much" by a broader culture or community. As driven, daring, and brave as they seem to be, Aries can be deeply hurt by this. After their natural instincts are criticized, they might learn to tamp down their fire, control the outward expression of their lust or longing, or to completely hide their natural volcanic eruptions of desire from potential or current partners—and even from themselves. But it's dangerous to cap a volcanic force. The more the natural Aries erotic instincts are forced underground, the fiercer the eventual eruption can be. This can come out in bursts of anger toward loved ones, or the Aries might turn their frustration back on themselves and become bitter and angry at the world.

I'll share a personal example that feels emblematic of this issue, since I am an Aries Sun sign (Chiron is also in Aries in my seventh house of relationships). At a junior high bat mitzvah, I'd spent the entire party badgering the DJ to play "Burning Up" by Madonna. The song is sexy as hell and has lyrics about being on fire and unquenchable desire. I know, could there be a better Aries anthem? Probably not, yet at the tender age of twelve, I had no clue. (Incidentally, it's an excellent sex soundtrack for both Aries and Leo seasons.)

The DJ finally played it when we were eating dessert and everyone was off the dance floor. The instant I heard the first bars, I jumped up with a mouth full of buttercream-frosted cake and DOVE OVER A BANQUETTE onto the dance floor in my blue taffeta dress, alone and undeterred. I began dancing wildly, doing the moves I'd practiced at home, falling to my knees and putting the back of my hand up against my brow during the chorus. Mind you—I had never been kissed, dressed modestly at school, and was basically a super nerd. This just happened unconsciously and instinctually. If I were a Leo like Madonna, I might've been doing it for an audience. But as an Aries, I did it simply because my body propelled me to.

After the song ended, I looked up. I was still alone on the dance floor, and all the parents were looking at me with horrified expressions. I blushed intensely, realizing that I had accidentally shown a part of me that wasn't meant to be seen. My excitement and yearning to dance was not meant for public consumption. The powerful shame stayed with me until my early twenties, when I lost my virginity to a very sweet boyfriend and discovered the power of my natural Aries sexual instincts, which eventually led to becoming a sex writer and clinical sexologist. (That song still gets me going every time, by the way.)

When their fire is put out by societally generated shame, Aries can appear flat, lifeless, cold, and bitter. That's the danger of pouring cement over that metaphorical volcano. I mostly channeled my repressed sexual energy into social justice causes during those years of internalized shame—so it didn't go completely to waste.

An Aries steeped in shame might not even want to *talk* about sex and desire, because they feel like it no longer *belongs* to them. Work must be done to reengage and reignite erotic energy if it once existed and was lost. Often, adult Aries have never truly met and accepted this part of themselves, because the environment they inhabited during childhood and adolescence shut it down before it could flower. But it's still there somewhere, just waiting for the striking of the match.

When Aries children are told that anger is bad, or that being overexcited and jumping up and down is too much, these little rambunctious Rams can get the message that their very *existence* is too much. Frankly, when not fighting a war or watching an MMA match, Aries energy can be something polite society would prefer not to engage with. Yet adult Aries are often naturally attuned to righteous rage, even when they're still working on developing a healthy sexuality. My advice is to honor the instinct to fight for what's right, even if you're still struggling to find the red-hot center of your sexual sovereignty.

## Aries Shame and Shadow Work

An Aries who hasn't done shadow work can be self-righteous, vain, and insecure in many parts of life, including in the sexual realm. A less aware Aries might start fights just to push people away—rather than bring them closer via healthy competition. Knowing the difference between a fun verbal joust and a damaging argument is vital to an Aries who wants to enjoy robust relationships and great sex. Watching actual Rams joust in the wild shows us how fine the line is between playfighting and deadly fighting—and an Aries must always be aware of this instinct within themselves, so as not to do any damage.

A repressed Aries might test people immediately upon encountering them, expecting to be met by antagonism even when none is present. They can project energy that feels bitter and angry rather than excited, passionate, and eager.

Because Aries must be in touch with their *primal instincts* to heal sexual shame, pursuing a healing journey through their direct relationship to their own body first can be very effective in helping them locate (or relocate) a hardy relationship with lust. Here are some examples of fire-generating tools I share with my Aries clients who wish to connect with their bodies more fully:

- Dancing is my personal go-to—simply turn on a favorite booty-shaking, pelvis-exploding song, dance hard, throw yourself around the room, and let yourself get turned on by your own movement. It may feel unnatural at first, especially if you perceive yourself not to have good rhythm, or to be a "bad dancer," but that's not what matters here. Feeling the music deep in your cells and allowing it to remind you that you're an animal—that's the work of meeting your Aries instinct. See what lights you up the way "Burning Up" lit me up as a tween.

- If dancing feels like too much, or you have physical limitations, watching *other* people dance can trigger the same part of your vestibular system. Follow dance accounts online—modern, hip-hop, salsa, pole dancing, and whatever else seems to wake up a connection to your own pelvic thrust.

- Masturbating even when you "don't feel like it." The key is to start slow. This is less about getting quickly to the moment of release and more about the journey. *Edging*, a practice often used in partnered sex to bring someone almost to the point of orgasm and then to slow down pressure or friction so that they come back from the edge of orgasmic release, can also be employed in solo sex. Try touching yourself as slowly and sensually as possible.

- You can also do a role-play between the parts of your body that feel fiery and the parts that feel bad. If your arms and shoulders feel lithe and fired up, but your pelvis feels locked or shut down, what can your arms teach your pelvis about becoming loose, yet strong?

After experimenting with any of these exercises with as much intention and attention as possible, try sitting down with your journal, once you've caught your breath, to capture what came up for you. If writing it down doesn't work for you, open your phone's voice app and record your answers.

## Journal Questions for Aries Shadow Work

- How often am I turned on during an average day, week, or month?

- If I am turned on, do I feel any residual shame about that state of arousal? What does it bring up for me?

- If I'm not turned on, do I feel any shame about that? Is there something underneath this feeling?

- Do any parts of my body feel resistant or numbed out?

- Do any parts of my body feel turned on or extra fiery?

## Gender, Patriarchy, and Their Intersection with Aries Sexual Concerns

Aries that have been socialized as women may carry shame about wanting sex in the first place. They may have been called sluts at an early age or accused of being oversexed by peers or partners. Although gender roles are a tricky issue in contemporary astrology, where we talk about "masculine" and "feminine" planetary energy, patriarchy seems to play a definitive role in the way that people of all genders express Aries energy. Those socialized as male are often more comfortable embodying Aries/Mars behaviors, especially aggression, physicality, willfulness, and the sheer and unadulterated confidence that a "man's man" is allowed to possess. In societies dominated by patriarchal systems, i.e., most societies, Aries men are often invited to be unconstrained. This can be dangerous and problematic, but at the same time, too much passivity can harm an Aries—regardless of gender identity, they have to find the proper balance. This is because inside, at some level, they will be raging against the dying of the light and moving to fight for what they believe in and what they lust for.

Aries humans socialized as girls and women, especially those from religious, conservative, or other more traditional backgrounds, can have a difficult time with these natural expressions of their sign's energy until they wholly, sometimes forcefully, un-shame themselves. Aries women barred from moving through the world at the breakneck speed of their souls can become depressed and angry and then turn that anger back on themselves. I feel lucky that I did this work in my early twenties, but I've had many clients who've moved through their lives without access to their Aries energy, and it always breaks my heart until I see them burst into flames and rediscover their birthright after a few sessions.

They can learn to feel comfortable setting the patriarchy on fire while *simultaneously* developing a positive relationship to the feats their body can accomplish, as this will free them to fully be who they are and express the full range of their desire. How? Perhaps by noticing the simple, invisible everyday gender inequities that have defined their lives or their love and sex lives. Do you want to dress louder? Do you want to wear red? Do you want to take up the space that's been denied to you? Do you want to skip when you walk down the street? Do you want to yell back at the catcaller who thinks they can get away with harassing you? If you're in a long-term relationship, does your partner get away with not doing any (or just less) housework or childcare? Demand time to allow your body to move without blowing up your relationship (unless you realize you *want* to blow it up). Like Libra, their opposite sign, Aries often need to chart a solo path before they can figure out who they are with other people. If you haven't done that, make it your business to figure it out.

By the same token, cishet Aries men must fight against the instinct to categorize their women partners, especially if Aries men have been raised in an environment rife with unprocessed toxic masculinity. Doing that work can create a major shift in power for Aries men—without making them feel smaller or weaker. In fact, when Aries men engage with this part of themselves, they often connect to a rich, untapped source of erotic power.

## A Deeper Look at Body Rulership
## and Erogenous Zones for Aries

The head, face, and hair are the ultimate Aries erogenous zones. Many Aries enjoy special attention to their faces, from the forehead, eyes and eyelids, the brows, the nose, the chin, the cheekbones, the earlobes, the scalp and skull, to the lips and mouth. (Aries shares the lips and mouths as erogenous zones with Taurus.) Temple and scalp massage, ear kissing and biting, hair-pulling, and running fingers through the hair can drive Aries over the edge. Whispers and dirty talk directly into or very near the ear are extra erotically charged for the Ram. Aries may love to drape their hair over their partner or to be draped by a partner's hair.

Spending extra time focusing on the erogenous zones is especially useful for Aries who often aim to get directly down to the business of intercourse. The same goes for solo sex. In solo sessions, an Aries may want to experiment with running their own fingers through their hair, massaging their scalp with fingers or a scalp massager, or pulling on their earlobes. Massaging their temples, jaw, and forehead gently or visualizing this can elicit immense pleasure.

## An Embodiment Exercise
## for Aries Season

### Fire in the Belly

Like Aries natives, this exercise is simple and gets right to the point.

You'll need a candle, an oil you're comfortable using on your face and in your hair, a yoga mat or rug, a towel, and your journal or phone's recording app for post-exercise notes.

Seated on the floor at the edge of your mat or rug, or whatever is comfortable for you, take a few deep breaths, holding your hands over your belly as you feel it expand on the inhale. Light the candle, paying attention to what the fire makes you feel, if anything. Stare at the flame or feel the heat of it for a few minutes and imagine the fire leaping over your head, flowing all the way down your spine and igniting your second or sacral chakra located in the genital region (see chakra diagram on page 19). Now add that visualization to your inflow and outflow of breath, with the flame descending with the inflow and rising with the outflow. As you breathe in, imagine the fire descending down your spine and into your genitals. As you exhale, imagine that it rises and releases above your head.

Keeping your oil in your hand, lie down on your mat, close your eyes, take a few more breaths into your second chakra, and apply some oil to your forehead. Gently massage your forehead, temples, cheeks, chin, lips, earlobes—let your hands go where it feels best, continuing your deep fire belly breaths. Feel free to run your fingers through your hair or massage your scalp, too. Do this for as long as it feels good, but aim to continue for at least ten minutes. If you feel yourself getting bored, retrain your attention to your fire belly breath, and change the position of your hands.

Do not be surprised if you get wildly turned on by this exercise, even though no genital touching is included. (This doesn't, of course, preclude you from masturbating afterward.) This exercise can be VERY activating, so find ways to get grounded afterward. Come into a state of relaxation and consider lying down in Savasana (Corpse Pose). This is a yoga pose in which you relax your whole body while lying on the floor with closed eyes, if that's comfortable, breathing normally. Aim to do this for ten minutes, and drink plenty of water after.

Bonus: this solo exercise can be modified for partner play. It's ideal for Aries season experimentation and extra hot if either partner is an Aries or has planets in Aries. Follow the same steps, but massage each other's faces and scalps in turn. Then see what happens next!

## Try These Tools to Connect with Aries Energy:

- When you feel yourself rushing, take a deep breath and slow down, or stop moving entirely, just for a few moments.

- Stay hydrated to control that fire without putting it out.

- Learn the nature of fire (safely). Have a conversation with a firefighter about what it feels like to control a blaze or explore the kink of fire play.

- Practice waiting your turn in conversations with lovers or those you might want to be your lover. Gently bite your tongue if you must.

- Pleasure a partner first, then take your turn.

# 3

# Taurus Sexuality

## Stillness and Sensuality

I want to do with you what spring does with the cherry trees.

**Pablo Neruda**

"Poem XIV: Every Day You Play"

**Dates:** April 21–May 21

**Sexual Archetype:** The Hedonist

**Motivation:** Pleasure

**Symbol:** The Bull

**Planetary Ruler:** Venus (also rules Libra)

**Element:** Earth

**Modality:** Fixed

**Erogenous Zones and Body Rulership:** Lips, Jaw,
Neck, Throat, Vocal Cords, and Thyroid Gland

Healthy Taurus energy is solid, strong, sensual, unswerving, grounded, pleasure-seeking, and effortlessly charismatic. Like a favorite rich food or another indulgence we crave, Taurus energy can be addicting, and if we can get comfortable with the idea of pleasure for pleasure's sake, there is no need to loosen the grip that sweetness has on us.

But when Taurus people get stuck in a sexual rut, fearing the transformation that can move their sexual/romantic/emotional lives forward, what used to feel good may begin to feel boring and stultifying.

### Senses Working Overtime: Taurus Season in Focus

In Taurus season we might find ourselves exhausted from the fiery output of Aries, ready to simply *be*, rather than constantly *do*. We're moving from cardinal fire to fixed earth, from urgency to stillness. This energy can feel like finishing a high-intensity workout, needing to simply sit for a few minutes, just letting your body sink into the floor, or moving from the active flow of a fast-paced Vinyasa yoga sequence to the calm regulation of Savasana (Corpse Pose). If we can imagine this, we can feel into what it means to go from Aries to Taurus season.

This midspring season is an opportunity for people of every sign to really understand what embodiment means. The stability of Taurus season is a feeling we can return to amidst the frantic pace of fire signs, the neurotic mental loops of air signs, and the intense emotionality of water signs. Here, in Taurus season, we are best equipped to meet our bodies on their own terms. During Taurus season, we might aim to imitate a lovingly tended cow, just chilling in a meadow, reveling in our own satisfaction. During Taurus season we can practice relaxing into being stroked, spooned, or maybe chewing some proverbial grass while lying in a bed of wildflowers, not doing anything productive at all with a lover or with nature as our lover. Taurus season is an ideal time to learn about ecosexuality, a movement and practice that is dear to my heart. This young and evolving activist art movement means different things to its adherents, but what strikes me as particularly Taurean about it is that allowing yourself to be turned on by nature is a major precept of ecosexuality. Sitting with your back against a tree, with its roots supporting you, running your fingers over the bark. Listening to the wind rustle the leaves. Sniffing the air redolent of a neighbor's rosemary bush. Simply watching the clouds float by with nothing pressing to attend to and filling up our senses with stimuli—ecosex practices are the perfect Taurus season non-activity activity. If you want to learn more about ecosexuality, read *Assuming the Ecosexual Position: The Earth as Lover*, by my friends Annie Sprinkle and Beth Stephens.

Taurus season is when we can indulge in pure, unadulterated pleasure with no regrets or shame or anywhere to get to on time. If we're busy, we might schedule in a few days of staycation, or at least a few hours if entire days don't seem feasible. Treating pleasure the same way we'd schedule errands, time at the gym, or lunch with a friend or colleague can be a leap, but it brings excellent rewards.

If Taurus season had a soundtrack, it would probably be neo-soul, dripping with sonic honey and unbridled sensuality. Taurus rules the throat and has a strong association with singing and singers. When I think of Taurus soundscapes, I think of the dulcet tones of D'Angelo, Erykah Badu, Maxwell, Victoria Monet, and Jill Scott—music meant for the slowest kind of seduction.

## Get to Know Venus, the Planetary Ruler of Taurus

Venus, known as the "Lesser Benefic," is connected with what is traditionally perceived as feminine energy. What do benefics do? They deliver pleasure—the things in life that feel good. Astrologically, Venus is associated with sweet, receptive, loving, soft, beautiful, and easy energy—a planetary lover, not a fighter. Chapter 14 outlines the inherent complexities in this planet in more detail. Ruling romance, fertility, and prosperity, Venus' domain covers many of the things we tend to covet. The Greeks knew her as Aphrodite, the goddess of love.

Assigned to Taurus, Venus is a natural beauty, deeply sensual, and connected to the landscape as much as the body. Assigned to Libra, Venus takes on intellectual airs and is concerned more with the concept of beauty rather than the natural world; think of fine art, refined aesthetics, and cocktail party chatter as an art form. Both kinds of Venus energy bring delight, but they come across quite differently.

I like to think of Venus as a radical, in the sense that seeking pleasure for pleasure's sake, also one of the directives of Taurus, upends the very notion of capitalism. One of my favorite books of all time, *Pleasure Activism* by adrienne maree brown, cuts to the core of what this means in theory and practice. Practicing pleasure is one of the ways we can take our bodies back, sensual experience by sensual experience, from a dominant culture that demands that our labor is sacrosanct. What if enjoying life for no reason at all, with no outcome attached—not because we're free after all our "hard work"—didn't make us feel shame but instead brought us joy and contentment?

Venus is the consort of Mars, the divine masculine archetype in astrology. Once again for the people in the back: all genders possess this energy, and this doesn't imply Mars energy is solely for those who identify with he/him pronouns. For those with strong Taurus signatures in their chart (this includes the Sun, rising, or other planets in Taurus), there is often a connection to the earthy, grounded side of the divine feminine. It's nurturing, sensual, and creates the sensation of safety and security. This energy can seduce us and invite us into a garden of earthly delights that feels deeply gratifying, and more than just a bit addictive.

## Taurus' Erotic Gifts

Sensorial satiation is the raison d'être for Bulls, and they're often okay with taking their sweet time getting there. When they are in tune with their best selves, savoring every sensation can be easier for Taurus people, and there is a lesson for other signs in just watching them live in their natural state. Taureans might exercise every one of their senses individually and intensely, while also able to access their other senses if the desire strikes. Giving all their attention to a single base note of a perfume can wholly define one moment, while the next might be taken up by the taste of an obscure spice. Even routine daily activities can provide intense enjoyment.

For a Taurus, eating is not just about hunger but about the taste of the food on every region of the tongue and overall mouthfeel, the sound of a crunch or squish, the scent of cooking, the colors and arrangement on the plate, and so on. And like eating, sex at its best is a whole meal, from deciding what to eat to collecting ingredients and cooking to devouring it bite by bite, all the way to dessert. A Taurus in touch with their erotic gifts will radiate sensuality, and that can be pretty damn alluring to potential partners. Unlike Aries, many Taureans prefer to be in relationships, and attracting partners can be easier for them than other signs, precisely because of their evident and unignorable erotic gifts. Taurus humans tend to have so much sensuality oozing out of them that others may notice it, even if a Bull has suppressed these instincts.

A healthy Taurus might inherently understand that because sensory input is everywhere all the time, sex is also a 24/7 affair. Whether partnered or solo, a Taurus in tune with this part of their soul can wake up and begin finding ways to engage in foreplay. The feel of the sheets against their skin, the sound of morning birds, or the first sip of hot coffee from a favorite chipped mug that feels just right when gripped with both hands—it's all erotic fodder.

I once dated a Taurus man who called me in the morning to tell me what he was going to buy and cook for me that night, and continued to update me through the day about ingredients he was adding. Once I got to his apartment, he insisted that I smell and taste the feast while I sat on the sofa drinking wine and listening to him regale me about his culinary skills, with a not-at-all subtle hint about what that might mean for me in bed. After a delicious meal that ended with a delicate chocolate mousse and freshly whipped cream, he happily provided that second dessert, and would not stop until I was fully satisfied.

That, in short, is why Tauruses can find themselves with ample dating pools.

The thing, though, about the aforementioned mug—it's probably the same mug that turned them on yesterday and the day before. Taurus thrives in stable situations, and once it finds something that works, they can stick with it for years and years, never tiring of the satisfaction it brings. Some might call this a rut, but this erotic gift is clear—at their best, they can extract pleasure from things that others find boring.

Healthy Taurus sexuality can also present as stamina—as in the kind of person who wants to stay in bed with a lover for hours and hours and hours. This might mean extremely extended foreplay, multiple orgasms, cuddling and kissing and caressing and pillow talk, and then yet another ignition of the sexual response cycle, from start to finish, expanding in concentric circles. Novelty is often less important for Taurus, as it just has to *feel good*. Taureans can become serial monogamists, choosing partners that remind them of the creature comforts of a previous lover.

Of all the signs, Taurus energy most closely mimics the pure energy of desire without affectations. When a Taurus lives shame free in their body, everything is related to their desire, even when they're not thinking about seduction or sex. "Too much is never enough," you might hear a Taurus mumble out loud. (Sagittarius is the other sign that vibes with this motto, but for more adventurous reasons.) Taurus humans can turn the act of wanting into an art form. The chasm of healthy Taurean desire is so deep it may seem to have no end at all. Yet even when they see someone or something they deeply desire, they probably know that waiting to touch them just prolongs the potential pleasure for both parties. And that's what they crave: pleasure that never ends. The erotic gift of a Taurus is not just that they *can* wait but that waiting itself can be an enormous, self-sustaining turn-on. The release of orgasm is sometimes not even necessary; it can feel that good to just keep going, and going, and going.

In the capitalism-steeped recent history of astrology, we often encounter tropes about Taurus and wealth, materialism, and luxury. I've never been comfortable with this. Although the "good life" is something we might associate with Taurus and its Venusian rulership, this doesn't require affluence. A culture that equates pleasure with luxury misses the point of living in a Taurus body, which is to say: a body that understands that pleasure is very, very simple and very, very necessary. Now, it is true that Taurus demands to be comfortable, and struggling with money is never comfortable. Part of the journey to healthy Taurus sexuality is figuring out how to be comfortable with the simplest version of what's right there in front of them, not an aspirational idea of something they don't yet have.

Value is a word often associated with Taurus, in the sense that their elevated taste and addiction to beauty make them an arbiter of exquisite standards. Yet the deeper insight here is that these values have nothing to do with money or the material world. Taurus brings us into a greater awareness of what we value and what we truly want and need.

## Pathway to Play and Creativity for Taurus

Taurus rules the throat, and self-expression is essential to access their erotic gifts. When their creative "song" is fully expressed and free-flowing, Taurus is better able to activate that first-thing-in-the-morning foreplay instinct—and make it last all day and night. Creativity is a large part of their erotic feedback loop, and all art forms are allowed, but get-your-hands-dirty creative outlets like pottery making, horticulture, and cooking often hit sweet spots. Reaching for hands-on, sense-activating artistic experiences is its own form of foreplay, no partners needed.

## Taurus' Erotic Challenges

The old trope about Taurus stubbornness is real, and it can get in the way of getting down to the business of pleasure. When fixed earth becomes less about fertile soil and more about getting stuck in the mud, desires that once satisfied can become habits that become fixations. The Bull can grow angry when pushed to shift their routine even in small ways, and this includes sexual routines. Their expectation is often that what once felt good will always deliver that shot of pleasure, but bodies change and lovers' needs can change, too.

Getting stuck in a repetitive sexual loop can eventually erode erotic pleasure. When we enter a room filled with fresh lilacs, no matter how delightful the scent is when it first hits our nostrils, the heavenly fragrance will fade within an hour. We may have to walk directly over to the flowers and put our face in its petals and take a deep inhale, or leave the room and come back to experience it anew. Even a Taurus, with their heightened senses, may eventually grow used to the same routine in both self-pleasure and partnered sex—especially with the latter.

Taureans cannot be easily pushed out of their comfort zone. They have crafted their routine over time based on what initially felt good and got their dopamine flowing. It may take years, but when that routine fails to deliver the expected amount of pleasure, Taurus humans may not react by seeking novelty. They might instead double down on their longing to restore the ecstasy they once knew.

When a Taurus is unable to exercise self-expression, emotionally or creatively blocked, or stuck in a loop of comfortable sameness, they can become depressed, angry, gloomy, and self-destructive. Their key phrase is "I HAVE" but it could just as easily be "I WANT"—and when they're left unsatisfied by sources of sensuality that once nourished them, discomfort can overwhelm them.

## Taurus Shame and Shadow Work

Taurus people are often shamed for being materialists or hedonists, sometimes both. There is a fine line between learning how to experience pleasure for pleasure's sake and knowing when too much is indeed enough. This is the kind of shadow work that a Taurus often has to engage in if they want to experience their truest sexual self and most exquisite erotic heights. In our sex-negative, body-shaming, consumerist culture, exploring these questions requires deep work.

As creatures of habit, Taureans are prone to getting stuck in rather legendary ruts. At its worst, this can look like compulsive hoarding, disorganized eating, substance use disorder, or unhealthy relationship attachments. Notice that I'm not including sex addiction here, because I don't use that outdated term. There just isn't a lot of data to support that sex addiction exists, beyond its media-hyped reputation "X celebrity enters rehab for sex addiction." However, I will sometimes refer to toxic or compulsive sexual behaviors instead. Although Taurus people can develop these tendencies, they're better known for sticking with one lover over a very long period, even when it's not working—sometimes to both parties' detriment. They are more concerned with holding onto what they have rather than exploring novelty. Once they've found something safe and pleasing, they're not commonly interested in expanding their repertoire—even after it stops feeling heavenly.

Taurus' opposite is Scorpio, and this polarity can be a key to understanding what makes the Bull tick. This shadow energy is rippling with transformational potential, and that can scare the Taurus, set in their ways as they are. This inherent fear of change speaks to the nature of their relationships. Even though they often prefer to be attached than to be single, partnerships can push them to places they wouldn't go on their own. And a Taurus really hates to be pushed. Sometimes we find a Taurus doing nothing, not because they're relaxing into the beauty and sensuality of the moment, but because moving feels like changing, and change is terrifying. But when they connect with a partner that can impel them to face change, they can grow by leaps and bounds.

Aneesha was a cishet Sun and Venus in Taurus woman in her midsixties who came to me after the end of a long marriage. She and her husband, Sadiq, had enjoyed a deep and fulfilling romantic and sexual relationship after they met in their late twenties and married at thirty-five. She described their first years together as an "unending honeymoon," especially because they didn't have children and had plenty of time to enjoy themselves. For the first fifteen years of their relationship, up until about the time she turned fifty, they had sex at least three times a week. At least once a week, they would go food shopping together, cook elaborate traditional Indian meals, and then have long sex sessions. One of the things that was so special about their connection is that they felt brave enough together to part ways with the conservative religious values of their families, forging their own path of pleasure together.

Sadiq, a Pisces, was most interested in their romantic and spiritual connection, whereas Aneesha could envelop herself in the sensation of sex and have multiple orgasms in missionary position. I remarked about how rare that is, and she explained that they had an excellent fit—the shape of his penis provided clitoral stimulation for her, a stroke of luck she considered a gift from god. She joked that this was where she found religion again. She described their sex as "totally vanilla and totally delicious." But as the realities of their changing bodies hit at middle age, they continued to have sex in the same way—and over time, it no longer felt good. Aneesha was experiencing menopausal shifts and genitourinary changes, but she would not get help or discuss them, even with her closest friends. Aneesha continued to crave touch and connection, and Sadiq wanted them to connect emotionally, but at some point, their lovemaking became so rote that they were both practically sleeping through it.

Rather than communicate her fear about the way her body was changing and do something about it, Aneesha shut down and turned away from Sadiq. As their sex life waned and finally fully evaporated, they never spoke of it and she turned to shopping for pleasure. She had never been particularly interested in fashion or materialism in general but was just trying to fill herself up with something that felt good.

When she came to see me a few months after their divorce was finalized, it was because she'd read an article about life after menopause and how women can "get their pleasure back" on their own. We began by making sure she was physically healthy—she saw her gynecologist and a pelvic floor therapist I recommended. We delved into the nature of the fears she experienced when her sex life with Sadiq began to break down. She admitted to me that "I just didn't want things to change." We began to explore experiences from her childhood when stability was lacking—she had lived in a house in the suburbs until her father had to move back to India for work when she was thirteen, and the family moved to a smaller apartment where she had to share a room with her sister. When she tried to share her feelings with her mother, she was shut down. That major and somewhat sudden change had made her crave stability in her relationship above all, even if it was stultifying.

We worked on helping her find the pleasure in her body again, and she learned to use a lot of lube, trying dildos of different shapes so she could experiment with insertion again, and clitoral stimulation using air suction vibrators at different speeds. At first, she balked, saying that she was used to "natural" sex, but when I suggested some home-play exercises incorporating aromatherapy before using her new toys, it was the beginning of Aneesha's return to pleasure. The last time I talked to her, she was beginning to date again, feeling secure about communicating with new lovers about her body and its needs.

The Scorpio shadow illuminates the fear of loss that can drive Taurus' need to hold onto people, things, and outworn habits that no longer serve their higher good. Fear of change, fear of death (even symbolic death), fear of the unfamiliar—what often stymies Taurus sexuality is this unrelenting refusal to accept that sensation must eventually transform.

Getting caught up in a pleasure groove is no reason to feel shame, but being aware of when too much of something is causing harm is a healthy habit Taurus people might want to develop on purpose.

## Journal Questions for Taurus Shadow Work

- What feels good to me?
- What has always felt good to me?
- What no longer feels good that I'm still doing, sexually and otherwise?
- What do I crave over and over?
- Do I want to break that cycle, and if so, how can I break that cycle?
- Where am I afraid of change?
- What small change can I make that feels safe for my body and doesn't interrupt my pleasure?

## A Deeper Look at Taurus Body Rulership and Erogenous Zones

Taurus rules the lips, jaw, neck, throat, vocal cords, and thyroid gland. We can better support healthy Taurus sexual energy when these areas of the body are given extra attention and even worship. This might mean something as simple as applying a soothing, flavored lip balm before bed every night, using a rich night cream on the neck and massaging and caressing that area, or using gua sha to stimulate healthy lymph flow. It might mean doing vocal exercises, the kind that professional singers do, each morning. It might mean deepening listening skills in order to be heard. It might mean asking the doctor to check thyroid levels and eating foods that nourish the thyroid.

During solo sex, this might mean paying extra attention to the lips, neck, and throat area instead of simply focusing on the genitals. Rich aromatic massage oils that are edible can be an excellent adjunct for

Taurus masturbation sessions, and great to have on hand for partnered sex as well.

Opening the throat and making space for deep listening and communication is essential for Taurus humans in relationships, but immense patience is required. A Taurus unable to use their voice may eventually become enraged or despondent. This can look like a scratchy throat, an inability to swallow, or the feeling of words getting stuck at the tip of the tongue. Being a good, patient listener and providing positive feedback is necessary. In relationships, centering communication is essential for all signs—but for Taurus it is the key to keeping that creative channel open and flowing. Using responses like, "What I hear you saying is . . ." and giving a partner time to respond can be transformational.

## An Embodiment Exercise for Taurus Season

### Finding Your A-Spot

This ritual engages the senses in the simple act of eating an apple. It's excellent for Taurus humans and healing for all signs to practice during Taurus season.

You can do a similar ritual with any fruit you favor, but the apple offers some sensory advantages, so it's an excellent starter fruit. The first time you do this ritual, try to be in a quiet space—turn off the TV and avoid background noise, if possible, because you'll want to listen to your body quite literally. This ritual can be done sitting or standing, but I'd suggest, for the first time, to sit comfortably and put the apple on a table in front of you.

Start by taking a deep breath and exhaling *ever* so slowly. Then take one slower inhale and exhale, because your first one was probably shallow. Maybe one more?

Now gently reach for the apple, noticing whether you're rushing. Are you grabbing the apple the way you grab your phone?

Pay attention to the sensation in your fingertips as it makes contact with the apple's skin. Is it cold? Room temperature? Slippery from recent washing? Pay attention to the way it feels in your hands, retaining your connection to the weight, shape, and slip or texture of the apple.

Now close your eyes, raise the apple to your nostrils, and take a deep inhale. Notice the different notes of scent. Press the apple against your cheek, forehead, or chest. Then open your eyes, pull the apple a few inches away, and examine its flesh, colors, indentations, the way the light shines on it. Now you're ready for your first bite. Close your eyes again.

Anticipate. Breathe. Don't rush. Raise it to your mouth, but before you do anything else, press it against your lips, and don't be afraid to lick it. Then open your mouth and take your first bite. What's happening? Are you hearing the crunch between your teeth? Does your tongue taste sweetness, tartness, a bit of both? What do you smell? Let the juices run down your face and resist the urge to wipe them away.

Take another bite with your eyes open. Does it taste different than it did when your eyes were closed? Keep taking bites this way, as slowly as you can. As you continue to eat, notice whether you feel satiated or if you're hungry. Notice any tackiness on your fingers, the aftertaste on your tongue and the roof of your mouth. Run your tongue over your lips and below your mouth—do you taste of sweetness? It's perfectly normal to get turned on during this ritual, and perfectly normal if you don't.

To fully experience our sexuality, we can all practice feeling into our bodies more fully. Taurus humans and Taurus season can teach us so much about embodiment: the way a healthy Taurus inhabits their own body conveys strength and solidity, no matter what shape or size they are. When they are willing to do their shadow work—and are grounded with their feet planted firmly on the earth that is their ruling element—they are pleasure incarnate.

## Try These Tools to Connect with Taurus Energy:

- As you move through your home, try to pick up the objects you need with more care, running your fingers over them, rather than just grabbing them.

- Engage your senses as often as possible. Leave Post-its around your house that say, "Take a sniff," "Listen to all the layers of sound," "Touch yourself," "What does such-and-such food taste like?" "Look more closely."

- Sit underneath a tree and see if you feel turned on.

- Eat slowly and chew every bite.

- Take extra time when you touch yourself or others.

# 4

# Gemini Sexuality

## Genius and Gesturing

I have nothing to declare except my genius.

**Attributed to Oscar Wilde**

**Dates:** May 21–June 21

**Sexual Archetype:** The Flirt

**Motivation:** Learning

**Symbol:** The Twins

**Planetary Ruler:** Mercury (also rules Virgo)

**Element:** Air

**Modality:** Mutable

**Erogenous Zones and Body Rulership:** Shoulders,
Arms, Hands, Lungs, and Nervous System

Healthy Gemini energy is sharp as a tack, swift as the wind, playfully quick-witted, dazzlingly brilliant, inventive, fast, flexible, and highly flirtatious. When at their best, natives of this sign seem to know *all* there is to know yet are always seeking more information. Learning to breathe while they inhale all that data can be a Gemini's biggest challenge.

A consummate talker who at their best also knows how to practice active listening, a Gemini can be a master communicator. This is an essential sexual skill that's not always easy to come by. It's worth repeating that our brains are our most important sex organ, and a Gemini brain may seem bigger than the rest—with room to grow. Yet their need for speedy synaptic circuitry can get in the way of their sexual satisfaction and intimate relationships, keeping them from lingering with what feels good, pushing them to seek the next shiny object. Gemini, as the sign of the Twins, is known for their duality, and their angel/devil dynamic can manifest in myriad situations. These two commentators are always in dialogue on a Gemini's shoulders, offering a variety of ways to think everything through. The secret here is that rather than opposing each other or acting as forces of good or evil, these twins are in a relationship—constantly communicating with one another, negotiating, and teaching the Gemini how to understand all sides of any potential argument.

## Listen like Thieves: Gemini Season in Focus

Gemini season greets us in the final month of spring in the Northern Hemisphere, when the fecundity of Taurus season has overloaded our senses and our minds are ready for a workout. Nature has completed its slow reverse striptease, and now the trees are dressed to the nines, covered in a canopy of wild green leaves and ready to party. The birds seem to be screaming, THIS IS WHAT WE'VE BEEN WAITING FOR! A cacophony of flora and fauna, Gemini season is *loud*, and we can tune into it by observing this symphony.

This midspring music begs us to leave the safe, comfortable confines of Taurus season, with its more rigid perspectives on love, lust, and relationships, and get outside into our neighborhood and beyond, where opportunities to meet, talk, and flirt with other humans may abound.

If Taurus season was about building a deeper relationship with our own senses, Gemini season is about expressing those sensual experiences and observations in a variety of languages, and potentially translating them to others. Communication and commerce are correctives to Taurean repose. Spring fever takes a turn during Gemini season from the body to the mind.

Moving from fixed earth to mutable air brings both movement and intellectual curiosity, where the world is yet to be discovered, analyzed, and talked about all day and night. The days are also getting longer, so there is more time to discuss our discoveries. Our circadian clocks are shifting too, and we might have more energy to stay up later to entertain riveting conversations.

All of springtime evokes the birds and the bees metaphor, but this is the time of year when birds seem even more frenzied with song and bees buzz almost frantically. Rachel Carson, author of *Silent Spring*, called this "the living music" of "insect orchestras." Gemini season can make us all into pollinators for whom talking, listening, and learning is the biggest turn-on of all.

## Get to Know Mercury, Gemini's Planetary Ruler

Gemini is ruled by Mercury, the Roman god of communication and travel—the Greek Hermes, messenger of the gods. Hermes was a *psychopomp* (a conduit for souls from the earth plane into the afterlife), and he was able to translate divine messages between worlds. This is likely one of the reasons Geminis are so entrancing: we can't look away from watching a divine messenger in action.

One cool fact about Mercury (Mercury adores facts) is that this is the only planet of the astrological pantheon that has been referred to with they/them pronouns—a planet that lacks a masculine or feminine gender assignment. Mercury aims to help us see all perspectives, in a hyperlogical "just the facts, Jack" sort of way.

Most of us know Mercury's traits because Mercury Retrograde phases are in all our feeds and on our radar three times a year. You may know that travel tends to go awry, emails are mislaid, and your phone or computer could go on the fritz. The interesting thing about Merc retro phases that no one tends to talk about is that the tech fails we experience generally come from human error, not inexplicable mechanical failure. In other words, it's people's BRAINS that are messing up because they're overwhelmed, distracted, or disinterested. Mercury, the Trickster planet, is constantly calling for a quickening, and during its retrograde phases, we can tune into the depth that's often missing from its stories.

## Gemini's Erotic Gifts

Gemini is the first air sign of the zodiac, and humans born under its influence often find it hard to hide their curiosity . . . about everything. In sexual or romantic relationships, this can be utterly captivating. And in fact, experimenting with an intricate verbal tango is often the way a Gemini entrances their own mind, leading to an onrushing of libido. In their element, Geminis often have a way of making potential and current partners feel like every conversation, from the lightest banter about pop culture to in-depth discussions about loving and being loved, is equally crucial. Geminis can entertain themselves, as one of their twins watches the other regale the room. And the better command they have of a conversation, the less anxious and more in control their sensitive nervous systems are likely to feel.

Why mention rooms full of conversation when discussing the erotic gifts of a Gemini? Because for this sign, the act of talking and listening can be deeply erotic. A healthy Gemini's flirting skills can be so well-honed they're able to drop a perfect bon mot into exactly the right place, sending waves of pleasure through their bodies. What seems like casual chitchat to another sign can be a primal, pivotal interrogation of desire for the Gemini, no matter what is being discussed. A potential partner may not even be aware that this is happening, and it really doesn't matter to the Gemini.

A healthy Gemini has learned to listen to lover(s) and remains ever eager to learn. Sex is less likely to grow boring over time, whether a Gemini is partnered or solo, simply because they're eager to learn and try new things, from new-to-market sex toys to fun positions to radical approaches to partnership. Learning about their attachment style by taking an online quiz or studying their current station on the Kinsey Scale can heighten and deepen eroticism for a Gemini, when for others, this might just be an exercise in abstraction. Sexuality is diverse and fluid across the lifetime, but of all the signs, Geminis seem to be most comfortable with trying out different roles and identities.

Active listening is their inherent erotic power. If they've developed self-awareness and are able to avoid distractions, a Gemini can tune directly into a lover's needs and follow instructions to a T. They're usually willing to study a map of the clitoris if their partner is a vulva-haver. They're probably willing to read a how-to about giving a great blowjob if their partner is a penis-haver. And even though they're not as tuned into their primal instincts like an Aries, or their sensual instincts like a Taurus, a Gemini will want to learn all the details, tips, and tricks about giving themselves ecstatic orgasms, too.

Because they're so good at multitasking, in sexual situations, healthy Geminis can deftly switch things up as needed, and stay in the flow. Their body rulership includes the arms and hands, and they tend to be skilled when it comes to the intricacies of touch. From touching a lover to touching themselves, they can get to the point quickly.

When they're in tune with their best self, Geminis are turned on by learning and always ravenous for information. Their brains seem to absorb more than other humans, and sometimes they appear like hungry baby birds for whom data points are food. Reading, listening to a podcast, learning a new skill—all these activities can bring a sudden wave of electric inspiration that opens a libidinous flow. This is a sign for whom facts are a form of foreplay. Because good conversations are usually a turn-on for Gemini people, sex can start at first text. Geminis can fluidly and flexibly entrance with their language skills. This can feel like a kind of magicianship—as a Gemini tells a story or recounts something they read that morning, unconsciously, there is an air of courting. When Geminis are alone, they may talk to themselves and laugh at their own jokes.

Speaking of jokes, one of Gemini's erotic powers is their inherent knowledge that sex is often funny—it doesn't have to be taken so seriously. Whether they're masturbating, making out with a partner, approaching orgasm, or briefly hanging out in the bliss of postcoital plateau (this is one sign that usually does not stay at this stage for long), a healthy Gemini knows how to have a laugh about it.

## Pathway to Play and Creativity for Gemini

As the cunning linguists of the zodiac, experimenting with language can unlock the deep and endless well of Gemini creativity. Gems are often called "players" pejoratively but truly—they were born to play with words. That might mean doing a daily crossword, writing poetry, freewriting each morning, writing erotica, and talking during sex. This might look like dirty talk or sweet nothings, but the key is to experiment. Talking to oneself during solo sex can also be mind-opening and open new erotic/creative pathways. The hardest experiment? Staying with one thing for an extended period of time. Geminis might not be able to stick with one form of self-expression for more than a few days, but even if it feels boring, they should try to stay with it a little longer. If this is an erotic journaling practice, for example, resisting the urge to abandon it in favor of another shiny object may be hard, but oh so worth it when they drop in all the way and find the golden thread that awakens the flashing neon billboard of their genius.

## Gemini's Erotic Challenges

If we think of Gemini's twins as a set of doppelgängers with different perspectives, one twin is usually delivering a message while the other may disagree or hear something that piques their interest, distracting them from erotic intimacy. If conversations are foreplay, a Gemini needs to stay focused and listen as much as they talk. But even if one side listens attentively, the other side might see something more interesting across the room, losing interest in the building erotic sensation in their body. This is why active listening is such an essential skill for Geminis.

Because they're not as deeply suffused with intrinsic sensuality as Taurus, their astrological predecessor, and a few other signs, a Gemini can suffer from getting stuck up in the airy ethers where bodies don't even need to exist, because the mind is keeping them busy. Overfocusing on intellectual rumination can activate a Gemini nervous system and flip the switch on their anxious energy, pushing the Gemini further away from embodiment and pleasure. As much as a Gemini can be the master of effortless-seeming repartee when they're confident, they can also descend into obviously nervous chatter, not letting other people get a word in edgewise. Their intimate conversations can go from charming to cantankerous. For Twinfolks, a balance must be struck between acknowledging that even though their brains are their most active erogenous zones, they must get out of their heads for long enough to feel into their other pleasure centers.

With rulership over the hands, Geminis can tend toward fidgeting. This sign also rules the lungs, so remembering to breathe deeply during erotic experiences, from start to finish, is essential. Gemini synapses can snap quickly, and they can lose track of the central thread of both conversations and their own orgasms. Mindfulness meditation can help in both cases, but especially the latter. Breathing techniques are one of the best tools Geminis can use on a daily basis—even multiple times a day— and during sex, all the way from first touch to orgasm. A few breathing practices are included later in this chapter.

A Gemini can present as a genius who can't make up their mind and wants to keep their options open. Sometimes, if a thus-far monogamous Gemini hits a sexual snag with a romantic partner, they might be quick to suggest opening up the relationship rather than getting to the root of the issue with their current lover—not as a healthy exploration of ethical non-monogamy, but as a means to escape the truer intimacy they may fear. In this way, they can miss an opportunity to learn more about their own needs and desires. Monogamy is certainly not for everyone, but if a Gemini (or anyone of any sign) has an inkling or curiosity about other relationship models, they should aim to have the full discussion with a partner early on. Gemini energy can feel like eternal teenager energy, and not everyone can keep up with this lively, can't-stop-won't-stop race to see, hear, and do everything.

## Gemini Shame and Shadow Work

As the sign most unfairly associated with being two-faced tricksters and dilettantes, Geminis can carry shame about how the world perceives them. They might assume that others see them as superficial and glib, and then act the part. These assumptions can make them trust themselves less and second-guess themselves more.

Geminis can often get away with skimming surfaces and changing the subject when they feel uncomfortable. Over time, this can become problematic, eventually making a Gemini quite nervous about plunging to their own depths erotically and in partnerships. This, in turn, can keep those they love or want to be loved by from noticing that they don't know everything about everything. Geminis, arguably one of the smartest signs of all, can carry shame about not being smart *enough*.

Gemini's opposite sign, Sagittarius, is the archetype of the philosopher, known to go deep into singular sources of wisdom, offering mega-sized doctoral-level analyses of cherished subjects. A Gemini is often so busy at the perception stage of experience that they can skip the next step—in-depth analysis—entirely. A superficial understanding of their own desires can cause them to pursue more frivolous love affairs, making it even easier to abandon partners when the lover gets too close, or perceives the Gemini too starkly. One of their secrets is that *they want to be the perceiver, not the perceived*. What Geminis might recognize as an aversion to boredom is often something a lot more complex. No sign fears intimacy quite the way that a Gemini can, because few signs fear knowledge of the *self* more than the Twins do. Constant movement can help them avoid these depths.

My client Jaimie was a nonbinary Sun, Mercury, and Mars in Gemini in their early twenties, just recently graduated from college and living back with their parents on Long Island while looking for a job in New York City. They had come out first as bisexual in junior high, meeting loving acceptance from their peers and parents. In their freshman year at college, Jaimie began to discover their nonbinary identity.

When they came to see me via Zoom at the height of the pandemic, they were feeling anxious, stressed, and agitated because, after a steady diet of serial monogamist relationships through college, each one lasting about six months, they were unable to date new people thanks to living at home during Covid. At first, Jaimie said their main concern was isolation and the sense that their sexuality was withering on the vine during what should be the best time of their lives. They were still managing to do a lot of flirting via DM, on multiple dating apps, and sexting, but it was not filling what Jaimie called the "heart chasm" in their life.

Jaimie had an amazing flair for words, telling stories at such a fast clip we often both became confused about their original point of departure, and it became clear that even though they'd come to me for help, they were still hiding. I began starting all our sessions with a shared breathing exercise to keep them grounded and on track. Jaimie soon told me they'd begin to masturbate with a fantasy of an ex-lover from college they fell for very hard and missed, but a few minutes into the fantasy, they'd become distracted by a sound in the other room, worried someone would hear them. They started putting on the TV so that all sounds would be muffled, but then they'd begin tuning into what was being said onscreen and their arousal would abruptly stop. They tried using porn on their phone instead, but were easily distracted from that. After a few sessions, they revealed that the main problem was that when they masturbated, they could not orgasm—and they were trying to make it happen at least once a day, becoming increasingly despairing over the lack of release.

Jaimie needed less stimuli, not more, and to feel safe enough to be truly alone and intimate with their own mind and body. I suggested doing some deep breathing and perhaps some simple meditation before masturbating, and to schedule it around the same time each day, rather than chaotically and randomly doing it out of boredom. Rather than using a sex toy to masturbate, I encouraged Jaimie to use their hand slowly and purposefully, and to consider using white noise in the background to muffle sound. I wanted them to proceed to pleasure from a calm state, so they could connect with a meaningful fantasy that would allow them to stay in the moment.

Finally, Jaimie broke down in tears in a session and told me that the sex in their relationships eventually felt much like their recent attempts to have solo sex: just when things got deep and emotionally intimate, they could no longer orgasm. Then they would bail from the relationship, sometimes entirely ghosting the partner they'd grown to care for. I told them that being under forced isolation was the best time of all to interrogate this tendency. Over the course of a year, Jaimie developed a deep, calm, loving intimacy with their own heart and mind, and by the last time we caught up post-pandemic, they were in a happy, healthy relationship with someone they met online, with no desire to break it off and run away.

By changing the subject over and over, breaking off a relationship immediately as a honeymoon phase begins to wane, or changing positions so many times during sex that their partners never get to stare into their eyes, Geminis can avoid the intimate secrets of their own psyche. Whether multitasking, keeping dozens of tabs open on their laptops, watching a YouTube video while the TV blares the news in the background, noise can be used as a way of avoiding what the quiet might reveal.

And a deeper secret: when Geminis acknowledge and work through their fear of being alone and empty of thought, they can master the entire universe, their relationships, and all the communication therein.

## Journal Questions for Gemini Shadow Work

- Am I afraid to be alone with my thoughts?

- What are my sexual secrets?

- If I imagine a conversation between my twins, what's the dialogue?

- What can't I stop thinking about?

- What am I avoiding?

## Bonus Writing Exercise: Emptying Your Brain with Your Hands

This exercise is something I've used with writing students and both astrology and sex coaching clients over and over again. It's particularly ideal for Geminis working on their shadows, and for people of all signs during Gemini season. It's a combination of the work of two of my favorite writers—a take on the Morning Pages ritual from Julia Cameron's *The Artist's Way* blended with a timed writing exercise from Natalie Goldberg's *Writing Down the Bones*. Many Geminis, even if they aren't professional writers, can get to the core of their shadow work when they tap their instinctive affinity for language.

Ideally, this exercise happens first thing in the morning, before any other activity. Pick up your journal and pen before you pick up your phone. Don't get out of bed or talk to your partner. Just open your eyes, open your journal, and begin the physical process of dumping your brain on the page for ten minutes without stopping. The key to this is that your hand must keep moving—it's a physical exercise as much as it's a mental one. Your pen moves across the page and doesn't stop. If you have to stop to think, you're doing it wrong. Rather than think, you simply write whatever comes to mind. It could be: "I have nothing to say; this is stupid. The paint on my ceiling is peeling . . .", or whatever seemingly dumb, meaningless thought drops from your brain, into your shoulder, arm, fingers, and onto the page. Remember, these parts of our body are ruled by Gemini.

Of course, first thing in the morning may feel impossible for you, so you can modify this exercise to write last thing at night, or if you get a break when, say, your infant is napping. Try to adhere to the other suggestions for this exercise, though, if you can't wake up and make it happen.

After ten minutes, you can stop. Try to do this writing practice consistently for at least two weeks. At first, nothing much may happen—all the words you produce could seem utterly pointless, and you might wonder why you're bothering. But as you train your brain for the Morning Pages dump, even after a few days, you might start recalling your dreams. A creative idea could spark suddenly, warranting further investigation later in the day. You could have a therapeutic breakthrough, allowing parts of yourself you've kept at arm's length to emerge from your deep subconscious and leap onto the page.

If you want to go deeper, you can use prompts for each writing session, perhaps the journal prompts in each chapter of this book, through the astrological seasons. Again, if you find that mornings don't work for you, you can use these prompts any time at all. The key is to time the writing and keep your hand moving—that's the only rule. Try, ideally, for ten minutes, but know that you can modify this to fit your needs, writing for a shorter or longer chunk of time.

## A Deeper Look at Gemini Body Rulership and Erogenous Zones

Gemini's association with the arms, hands, and fingers gives it a readiness for play. Geminis often have long arms and attractive fingers. Even if they don't appear this way at rest, once they're witnessed in motion, it's almost as if they've learned a choreography, as if they're playing an invisible piano or typing on an invisible keyboard. The hands and arms often appear to flutter like hummingbirds, always buzzing around in motion. A lot of Geminis gesture wildly, throwing their hands around for emphasis.

Geminis are often skilled at crafts that require dexterity—from video games to knitting to plucking chords on a guitar to using their fingers to find exactly where a lover's pleasure point is to get them off with speed and ease.

A Gemini's arms and hands are very often deeply sensitive, especially the inside of the forearm and the palms. They can enjoy having their fingers stroked and sucked, and tend to love both gentle and vigorous hand massages. A lover's fingers gently tracing the inside of the shoulder blade, down the upper arm, wrapping around the forearm and down to each finger, one by one, can be powerfully erotic for a Gemini. And when solo, Geminis can play with their own bodies this way, as a prelude to genital stimulation or just to activate their erogenous zones.

## An Embodiment Exercise
## for Gemini Season

### Arousing Active Stillness

Sit cross-legged or on a chair with your feet on the floor or in whatever sitting position is comfortable, with your hands open on your knees, if possible. Close your eyes if this is comfortable for you and chant OM (the sacred traditional Sanskrit sound that symbolizes the essence of supreme consciousness in the Hindu tradition), or choose any word that feels meditative to you and repeat it three times. Perhaps your word is *love*, or *mmm*, or really anything at all. Take four slow, deep breaths, in through your nose, down to your sacrum, and rising up your crown chakra, visualizing that you're breathing in pink light and exhaling any excess stress or shakiness out through your nose. As you breathe, notice where your breath is holding or catching, then tune into the energy from your feet to the top of your head to identify any areas of tension, weakness, numbness, heat, or cold. This is a kind of active stillness; it's not complete relaxation, although it may feel relaxing.

I recommend trying this for ten minutes, if you can, but any length of time is beneficial. As you sit and breathe, visualize sending white light to any stressed areas of your body, washing them with cool, sweet Yin energy. In traditional Chinese medicine, Yin energy is cold, wet, and earthy—it's thought to be grounding. See this Yin energy as pale or pink light traveling up and down your spine, if you're not bathing specific areas of your body that need attention. When you're finished sitting in stillness, slowly bring your focus back to the room around you, perhaps opening your eyes and stretching out into a restorative Savasana (Corpse Pose). What this might look like: lie on the floor with your feet a few inches apart, your arms at your sides, palms facing up.

Close your eyes and soften the tissue of your face and skull. You can finish this exercise by gently massaging your arms and hands, after you've rested for a bit, while still lying down. You might tune into whether or not you're feeling aroused and see what you feel like doing with that information.

## Try These Tools to Connect with Gemini Energy:

- Begin the day with a simple breathing exercise in bed, inhaling through your nose, counting to five, then exhaling through your mouth slowly while counting to five. Repeat this five times.

- Practice deep listening in simple conversations with people you encounter during your daily errands, focusing on what they're saying and waiting to respond until you've breathed deeply for a few beats.

- Regularly use hand cream that you enjoy, and massage it sensually into your hands and arms before bed.

- If you struggle with certain meditation modalities, try different kinds of meditation, like walking meditation, adult coloring books, or tai chi.

- During sex or arousal, gently remind yourself to breathe deeply.

- Tell yourself jokes out loud when you feel anxious and let yourself laugh raucously.

# 5

# Cancer Sexuality

## Intimacy and Interiority

I stayed under the moon too long.
I am silvered with lust.
Dreams flick like minnows through my eyes.

**Marge Piercy**
"Moonburn"

**Dates:** June 21–July 21

**Sexual Archetype:** The Protector

**Motivation:** Nurturing

**Symbol:** The Crab

**Planetary Ruler:** The Moon

**Element:** Water

**Modality:** Cardinal

**Erogenous Zones and Body Rulership:** The
Stomach, Breasts, and Lymphatic System

Healthy Cancer energy is warm, soft, supple, nurturing, intuitive, emotionally attuned, highly sensitive, and equally sensitive to other people's needs. At their best, Cancers ride the tides of their love and sex lives without feeling like they're drowning. As emotionally vulnerable as they can be, tapping into a sense of their own sexual security can be their biggest erotic challenge.

Crabs are creatures that live in a watery liminal space: the border between the deep ocean and dry land. In this way, Cancers are often deeply contemplative and ardently relational, constantly figuring out where their own feelings end and a lover's emotional life begins. In ideal conditions, when shame is held at bay and safety and security needs are met, Cancers can reach heights of pleasure that other signs struggle to connect with. Once they give themselves over to it, a kind of hungry hedonism can take over. Like a cranky baby who has finally learned to latch to their mother's breast or an adult filling their belly with sustenance, a Cancer that gets a taste of soul-soothing eroticism may not know how to stop suckling.

## Summertime Sadness: Cancer Season in Focus

Coming off the speedy and chaotic high of Gemini season, we meet the season of the Crab on the longest day of the year in the Northern Hemisphere. As the Sun enters Cancer on the summer solstice, we're instantly enchanted by oceanic magic, even if we are far from the sea. We might tune into this watery magic at a lake, river, or even a backyard or local town pool. But if we are lucky enough to be near it, we can feel the seabirds and crustacean creatures responding to the solar/lunar vibe shift. And subconsciously, as we spend more time under the summer nighttime sky, even if we're doing so at backyard barbecues or chilling on rooftop bars, we might sense into eternal cosmic mysteries. Time spent under moonlight and starlight will do that to you—make you wonder about stellar origins or your own.

When we are close to the sea, the waves tell an emotional story as they ebb and flow and crash on the shore. We might tune into the phrase, "I'm all up in my feelings," in a very palpable way. Even if we are playing outside, part of us may turn inward. This is that quintessential "summertime sadness" that Lana Del Rey sang about so beautifully.

In Cancer season, we can feel into our own mysteries and more specifically, our own sexual mysteries. We might ask ourselves: Where did our desires take shape? How did our longings begin? What were we born with and what have we acquired? The lunar rulership of this sign makes late June and July nights feel mystical and almost eerie, as if we're suspended in a dream state. When we remember the summers of our childhoods as one long, endless stretch of unstructured days, it can feel like we're remembering a dream. In Gemini season, we get busy collecting data and perceiving our environment, and Cancer season is our chance to factor in our feelings.

Even though summer is the second season of the year and Cancer can be considered the moody teenager of the zodiac, Cancer season's association with mothering and wombs can feel like being born again or giving birth into a comforting, temperate sea. Wombs are deeply associated with this time of year. After touring fire, earth, and air, our seasonal experience of cardinal water can make us crave creature comforts and memories of safety and nourishment.

Somehow summertime brings many of us back to our childhoods, no matter our age, especially if we spent some of those young summers near a body of water—even an inflatable pool in our backyard. The association of the summer solstice with markers of "schools out for summer" and the freedom of endless days is imprinted on memories of adults who get no such seasonal break from responsibility. But even grownups tend to delight in ice cream on hot July days, and parents enjoy taking their kids for sticky-sweet cones, often for their own secret nostalgic reasons. (I have never met a human who doesn't like ice cream, so if you are that person, I apologize for not being inclusive.)

Sticking with the ice cream metaphor to better understand Cancer season as the start of summer, we might look at it like this: in Aries season we see an ice cream truck and rush over to it to grab a cone. In Taurus season we close our eyes and let the creamy deliciousness overtake our entire body through our tongue. In Gemini season we share a cone with friends or lovers and talk about how this is the best ice cream shop in town, almost forgetting to eat it. In Cancer season, we remember all the times we've loved ice cream before and try to replicate those experiences in the current moment.

In this way, the cacophony of Gemini season gives way to a feeling of returning to something that almost feels preverbal. Sometimes during Cancer season we experience an inability to articulate quite what we're feeling, because there is just so much emotion.

The Moon, Cancer's ruler, is the celestial body that knows the score: it functions as a memory bank for us in this way. We don't consciously remember being in the womb, but somewhere in our body-mind those sense memories remain—this is the domain of the Moon. In Cancer season our relationship with the Moon can deepen, as we're more likely to be out under it during warm summer nights. This is another way of saying that our instincts are alive now, and having access to these instincts is key to understanding ourselves as sexual beings.

## Get to Know the Moon, Cancer's Ruling Luminary

Looking at the Moon—whether it's full or just a slim Cheshire smile shape—can feel like an incantation. We don't need to do anything, or to make a wish. The Moon is just there for us, hanging in the sky, almost close enough to taste, unlike the planets that require astronomical knowledge or a telescope to find and recognize. The Moon's presence feels unlike the harshness of the other luminary, the Sun—a body we can't even look at directly without harming ourselves. The Moon gives us the gift of letting us gaze upon her whenever the sky is cloudless and her cycle provides a glimpse. The wonder of this is that it happens over and over again, endlessly—if we miss it, we will get another chance soon enough.

The Moon travels the entire zodiac in twenty-nine days and enters a new sign approximately every two-and-a-half days. This is a helpful way to understand the constantly shifting moods of Cancer humans and Cancer season. Not only does the Moon move between signs, taking on each sign's personalities and emotional qualities, but it makes aspects to other planets along the way. Cancers seem to feel all of these, like the proverbial princess in "The Princess and the Pea," constantly ebbing and flowing into various feelings. During Cancer season, we can invite ourselves to be in the world like this, no matter our sign.

The ebb and flow of the sexual response cycle, from desire to arousal, plateau, orgasm, and resolution reminds me of a lunar cycle, which flows from the New Moon, waxing crescent, First Quarter, waxing gibbous, Full Moon, waning gibbous, Third Quarter, and waning crescent. Yet within both the sexual response cycle and the lunar cycle, there is variation. The Moon will always wax and wane, but it will start at different degrees of different signs from month to month. Our sexual response cycles will also wax and wane over the course of our lifetimes, our relationships, and even from one day to the next. This shows that there is no wrong way to feel—the Moon only tells us that we must feel *something*.

The Moon seems to know us best, perhaps because it's the closest and most familiar object in the solar system to the Earth, like the old neighbor who lives a few doors away and watched us grow up, coming and going and growing and playing and crying as we entered and left our own house. The home is one of Cancer's most sacred spaces and an essential metaphor for understanding Cancer.

Astrology memes about Moon-ruled folks building their sacred womb-rooms, not wanting to leave the house, and being hygge (the Danish art of coziness and comfort) experts tend to ring true for many Cancers, even those who enjoy a nice social outing. Having a safe space to retreat to when the world gets to be too much—where the Cancer or Moon-ruled person can safely emote without judgment—can feel essential. Many kids like to build forts and caves to hide in, but Cancers can long for the sensation of being swaddled and protected deep into adulthood.

### Cancer's Erotic Gifts

The endless well of Cancerian sensitivity is both the Crab's erotic gift *and* their challenge. This sign leaves nothing on the table. Cancers tend to feel *everything*, which is to say they can be enveloped by the experience of pleasure with their entire mind, body, and soul when conditions are right. This sign can ripple with ecstasy from the gentlest, most wispy touch from a lover, particularly when their feelings are strong and they feel safe. Full body orgasms are possible, as are nipple-gasms, since Cancer rules the chest and breasts.

We often use food metaphors when we talk about Taurus, the sign of the five senses. When Cancers are in touch with their erotic gift, they are attuned to the art of feeding and being fed. This is a metaphor that goes far for Cancers—when food itself enters the bedroom, it can enhance or become the entire focus of a sexual encounter. This can be something as simple as preparing or sharing a delicious meal as an act of foreplay, or of being naked with food, having food eaten off the body, inserted in orifices, and so on.

The Moon is the sensorial connective tissue here, with its dominion in Cancer and exaltation in Taurus, giving Cancers sensitivity to pleasure that might feel familiar to someone with Taurus placements. Cancers can immerse themselves in sensory pleasure as fully and wholly as Bulls can, but the difference is that where Taurus can give themselves over just because it feels good, Cancer usually needs to have a deep emotional connection—even for just one night. Both signs can immerse themselves so fully into pleasurable experiences that it can look like pure hedonism to outsiders, but Cancer's little secret is that their pleasure hinges on getting their security needs met.

When a Cancer feels safe and held, they'll often let the soft animal of their body (thank you, Mary Oliver) out of its protective shell, and ecstasy can then ensue. This is when they can give themselves fully over to the experience, and where their sensitivity only heightens their pleasure. The touch of a lover or of their own hand or a sex toy can send their body into a paroxysm of delight even before they orgasm. Without the shell, every brush of the skin, every movement, every moment their eyes meet a lover's eyes—it can all feel like being extremely high.

This sensitivity extends to Cancer's visceral intuition about their lover's needs and longings. When they're at their sexual best, unbound by fear and shame, they can anticipate a partner's desire before it's expressed, and often before their lover even consciously knows what they want. Even though Cancers are superficially known for their shyness, being naked in all ways with a lover who makes them feel secure brings them right out of their shell.

The Cancerian circle of trust is a very special place, and their sexual circle of trust even more so. Creating and nurturing a safe, healthy container in which to experience the pleasure of emotionally fortifying erotic connection, even to their own body, is what Cancers deserve and can achieve with practice.

## Pathway to Play and Creativity for Cancer

Just as the Moon illuminates the night sky, giving us a code to understand the darkness or the parts of our subconscious that are unknown to us, Cancer's pathway to play is an invitation to go within. Tapping into the silent spaces in the subconscious and opening the instinct and intuition to all the creatures that come out at night is one way to open this creative door. Dreams are a vast resource—keeping a journal at the bedside and writing down images, ideas, and emotions from the previous night can offer a rich, fertile, creative option. Playing with memoir—writing the story of one's life, either in snippets or chronological order—invites the lunar reflection Cancer craves. There's a lot of material to be mined, erotic and otherwise, by digging into ancestral roots, whether with a DNA kit, a box of old photos, or conversations with family elders.

## Cancer's Erotic Challenges

It's that sensitivity again—this is where Cancers can experience their greatest erotic challenges. Building their circle of trust, one that leads to healthy, safe, loving sexual relationships, is often full of starts and stops. Getting their security needs met is essential, and yet most non-Cancer humans don't relate on that wavelength and may call out their Cancer partners for being too "needy," causing a shame spiral.

The tendency toward a codependent attachment style is common here, as Cancers might spend their adult lives searching for someone who will mother them as fiercely as they were mothered (if that was a positive experience) or trying to re-parent themselves after struggling with poor or incomplete parenting. They sometimes turn to those who seem to need even more than they do in order to make sure they'll always be needed. Clinging to familiar and safe people and spaces can create codependent relationships that have lost their sexual luster but feel secure. Cancers will often choose sexual relationships where they can assign themselves the task of taking care, sometimes even financially, in exchange for being with someone whom they perceive to be tolerant of their sensitivity. When I meet a client with prominent Cancer placements, one of the metaphors I use with them is "it feels like all your organs are on the outside of your skin." There is a deep well of sensitivity that is unmatched, and sometimes it hurts so good that Cancers need to retreat into their shell for protection.

Nourishment is necessary here, but the shadow side of this is starvation. For Cancers, this might mean attending to the bodily need for nourishment quite literally—eating delicious food regularly throughout the day, not letting themselves get too hungry between meals, and making this into a kind of ritual. This may also mean nourishing the spiritual and emotional self every day, in small ways that are replicable and simple.

When a Cancer isn't facing the enormity of their feelings or they're isolated from caring connections, they can experience disordered eating. Regular routines that remind a Cancer of the ebb and flow of the Moon-ruled tides can also help them with emotional regulation. A morning cup of coffee or evening cup of tea in a cozy spot near a window, where they can sip slowly and enjoy the light changing through the seasons, is but one way to remind themselves of the cycles within their bodies that are replicated in nature.

The Cancerian erotic nature may be naturally self-protective, as they sometimes fear exposing their soft, vulnerable interior to rejection—an emotion that might feel like a dangerous predator. Walking sideways can help them avoid getting caught up in unhealthy love affairs and toxic sexual situations, as they survey and test potential lovers before giving them their everything. This might mean taking things slow at first, spending a few weeks texting or talking on the phone leading up to meeting in person (especially when they're doing online dating). It could mean having an upfront conversation about their need to regularly take space, so potential lovers don't assume they're being rejected.

## Cancer Shame and Shadow Work

The Cancer shadow can be both controlling and controlled, in possession of structures that prevent it from becoming overly emotional.

Saturn, the ruler of Capricorn, Cancer's polarity, rules the bones, but Cancer only has a shell—it's not as strong as a bone. Often, even within their shell, Cancers feel too soft to survive predators or the elements. Cancer shadow work can require an interrogation of the ways they hide themselves or sidestep their emotions in order to avoid drowning in them. Finding that balance between hard and soft, unfeeling and feeling too much, is the way Cancers eventually create enough safety to immerse themselves in their mystical inner world, where they have access to ecstasy whenever they want to tune into it.

One of my cishet male Cancer clients struggled with his sex life well into his late thirties. As a serial monogamist who only wanted to find his one true love, Stuart kept choosing younger women who struggled with money. But even though he had not yet "made it" himself, at least he could offer them something, he told me. It was an "I feed you, you desire me" kind of exchange for him.

With women like this, Stuart felt sexually self-assured, at least at first. After months had passed and he felt more emotionally exposed—having cried in front of his partner, in one case—he would shut down sexually. His libido decreased as soon as his partners developed more autonomy. One lover got a new job and no longer needed him to help her with rent, and he soon found himself experiencing erectile issues with her. Rather than facing his fears and shame, he ended the relationship.

This happened two more times with other women he met at his IT job. In one case he even encouraged his partner not to take a promising job at another company so that he could continue to financially assist her, an unconscious bid to extend the cycle of his sexual prowess. He wondered if there was something medically wrong with him, but after a urologist assured him he was healthy and gave him a Cialis prescription, he used that to mask his emotions for another year. Getting erections, he thought, was all that mattered. Eventually his ED became DE (delayed ejaculation), and that's when he booked a session with me.

When I saw his chart, I asked about the financial dependencies, and whether he thought they had anything to do with his sexual issues. He began to cry and revealed that he didn't know how to be with someone without taking care of them first. We focused on how Stuart might first begin caring for himself, tending to his own needs, both erotic and financial, and when he eventually began dating again, he set boundaries around doing too much caretaking. This completely changed the way he engaged with his partners sexually. After six months, he was once again in a monogamous relationship, but this time with a partner who didn't need him as his previous ones did, neither financially nor in other ways. Keeping communication open about his fears and vulnerabilities was a huge part of his journey to feeling safe and empowered in bed with his lover—someone he felt safe enough to cry with, and to hold and be held by.

If we want to talk about Cancer shadow work, we also have to talk about mothers and mothering. Regardless of gender, the mother archetype is embedded in the Cancerian imagination. Whether a Cancer is a devoted mother or plans to become one, dearly loves or has a complicated relationship with their mother, loves the mother of their children or is estranged from that person, is a guardian of children but not a mother, or is childfree by choice, the MILF (Mom I'd Like to Fuck) or Bad Mom acronym often looms large.

Many cultures fetishize mothers in unhealthy ways (we could spend a whole book talking about the patriarchal implications of the virgin birth). In line with this, Cancers often find themselves longing for sexual satisfaction that matches this fetish, whether they want to be adored and worshipped like a mother goddess or want to do that worshipping at the altar of a lover. This can sometimes create unhealthy or even toxic relational patterns for Cancers. Often this goes both ways, as the more care they give, the more reciprocal care they want to receive, even if they won't say it out loud.

Even though slipping back into a hard shell creates the illusion of safety, it can shut Cancers off from discovering the full depths of their sexual selves. Facing their shadow—a side of them that might be overly controlling and domineering—can help them discover the deep sea of their sexuality, rich with pleasures that aren't necessarily bound to codependency or unrequited love or lust.

## Journal Questions for Cancer Shadow Work

- How do I feel held?

- Who or what am I holding onto in order to feel held?

- What kind of touch makes me feel nurtured?

- What do I miss about past versions of me? What do I miss about the sexual being I once was?

- What anchors me in the safety of my body?

## A Deeper Look at Body Rulership and Erogenous Zones for Cancer

Cancer rules the chest and breasts, and natives, regardless of gender, might be obsessed with breast stimulation and nipple play. It's often said that everyone loves breasts, but Cancers might love them more—or have a complicated relationship with them.

Although breasts and nipples are common erogenous zones for all signs, Cancers often have extremely sensitive breast tissue. This can be very pleasurable, but sometimes this sensitivity is overwhelmingly intense. If this is the case, experimenting with gentle touch, light licking, and soft fondling can be a bonus for Cancers and their lovers.

Cancers may want to engage in admiring, fondling, caressing, kissing, and sucking partner's breasts, sometimes to the exclusion of touching other parts of their body, for exquisitely long periods of time—or to have their own breasts treated this way. Breast and nipple-gasms are possible for the Cancer or their lover, and this kind of experimentation can be loads of fun for all.

If sensitivity to pain is not an issue, bondage gear focused on the breasts could be fun to play with, so an investment in nipple clamps might be warranted. On the other hand, suckling skills can give a Cancer some serious talent when it comes to providing oral pleasure to a partner (cunnilingus, blowjobs, or analingus equally). There can be a sweetness and tenderness in the way Cancers perform these sexual acts.

# An Embodiment Exercise
## for Cancer Season

### The Erotic Moon Gaze

Allowing ourselves to be bewitched and erotically enriched by the energy of the Moon can make our own sexuality less mysterious to us during Cancer season, or anytime we feel like connecting to our own emotional body. Like in the Taurus chapter, this embodiment practice is drawn from my work in the ecosexuality movement.

How far you go with this exercise will depend on where you live and what kind of outdoor space you have access to, but it's an endlessly modifiable practice, so experiment wildly with it. This can be done alone or with a partner, or even with a group of like-minded Moon-curious folks.

You can try this even when the Moon is new and less visible, but the first few times you practice it, you may want to choose the days after the Moon begins to wax, preferably when it is full or within three days of being full.

Prepare a small portion of any food or drink you find comforting and nutritive to bring with you. Wear loose, comfortable clothing, and if you have privacy and feel comfortable, clothing that you can quickly and easily remove. Aim to choose a cloudless or partly cloudy night and wait until about two or three hours after the sun sets to go outside. Choose a spot where you can gaze at the Moon unobstructed by tall buildings, large trees, or other barriers between you and the night sky, like a rooftop if you're in a city.

This ritual can be performed standing or sitting—but you must have a view of the Moon.

Start by tuning your focus upward, perhaps closing your eyes, taking a deep breath, and becoming aware of your body to see where you're holding any tightness or discomfort.

Notice if you have any intrusive thoughts. Notice where you are on your own arousal continuum—are you feeling anything you would describe as desire or horniness?

Now tilt your head to the sky and open your eyes if you closed them. Drink in the Moon with your eyes if you can, and then try to add the rest of your senses one by one. Is the Moon whispering anything in your ears? You may hear other outdoor sounds as well.

Take a deep inhale of the air, like you're a wolf about to bay—what does the air smell like? Of course, we can't literally smell the Moon (maybe one day!), and you may smell trees or something unpleasant like garbage, but just for the sake of this exercise, assume that everything flowing into your nostrils and other senses is of the Moon's essence.

Now take a bite or sip of the food/drink you've brought with you, nurtured by the essence of the lunar energy, as if the Moon itself is serving you what you love.

Close your eyes again, reach up toward the sky if you can, pulling the lunar energy toward you, and if it feels good to you, run your hands over your belly and breasts/chest. Now it might matter where you are—whether in a public or private place. If you're with a partner, you can run your hands over yourself first, and then each other. You can do this as many times as you want.

What are you aware of in your mind and memory now? Tell the Moon. Whisper your secrets, or speak them boldly. Listen for a response.

Now do a second body scan. Which part of your body is lit up? Has the earlier tension eased? What instincts have kicked in? Have any desires emerged from the depths of your subconscious? What has been illuminated?

## Try These Tools to Connect with Cancer Energy:

- Learn where the Moon is at all times: install a Moon phase app or get a Moon phase notebook.

- Spend time by the sea or another body of water.

- Try daily breast, chest, or belly massage with essential oils.

- Witness and greet the Moon as often as possible, even just by peeking out the window if it's inconvenient to go outside.

- Care for yourself at the exclusion of anything else on your to-do list.

# 6

# Leo Sexuality

## Play and Performance

> The play's the thing.
>
> **Shakespeare**
> *Hamlet*

**Dates:** July 21–August 21

**Sexual Archetype:** The Lover

**Motivation:** Vitality

**Symbol:** The Lion

**Planetary Ruler:** The Sun

**Element:** Fire

**Modality:** Fixed

**Erogenous Zones and Body Rulership:** The Heart,
Back, Major Arteries, and Thoracic Spine

Healthy Leo energy is hot but not bothered, casually confident, impossible to ignore, dynamic, creative, playful, and ardently expressive. When at their best, Leos unflappably take and hold center stage, and their fans (better known as friends and lovers) are happy to revolve around their glamorous, star-bright presence. Yet when they become addicted to the dopamine of ego-stroking or worse, live an uncreative life, they can face their biggest sexual challenges.

What does a Leo want? If we see Leos through the lens of their animal totem, the Lion, the obvious answer is they want to be stroked. But it's their ego that craves caressing, not necessarily their mane. Leo, as the second of three fire signs of the zodiac, loves to blaze, yet as a fixed sign, it sustains its fire a bit longer than Aries. Think of this like going from a lit match or a firecracker to a mesmerizing all-night bonfire on a beach.

Leos, like all fire signs, are often instinctually and effortlessly powerful sexual beings. Yet where an Aries might burst forth like an arrow of throbbing, uncontrolled, forward-marching desire, Leos tend to glow hotly, magnetizing whatever they want. In this way, they might appear slightly lazy, like a cat dozing off in a warm ray of sunshine or a royal served by their court, blissfully enjoying what they know they deserve. But even the kind of Leo that expects to be cuddled and coddled can have a pure and feral hunting instinct when it comes to erotic endeavors.

## Sunshine of Your Love: Leo Season in Focus

When we meet this midsummer sign, it's hot outside. Think of a Lion less as a predator here, but as a large, playful animal rolling on its back with its belly showing. A healthy Leo knows they're the ruler of the jungle so they can relax and have fun. The roar is just a matter of projecting their voice through whatever theater they're commanding.

As we turn from Cancer to Leo season, we move from introversion to extroversion. We glide from uncertain, tilting tidal waters to the hot center of the beach, where we can lay out our towel, put on a pair of chic sunglasses, slather on the SPF, and worship the Sun, Leo's planetary ruler. After swimming in our unconscious watery depths and relentlessly feeling all our feelings for the last month, we're ready to celebrate and indulge in the art of play. Leo season is the corrective for the unswerving inward gaze of Cancer season, with its navel-gazing and endless emoting and processing of feelings, as necessary as that is. The Moon may have been a harsh mistress at times, but now it's more than alright to have a good time.

And as the Sun changes position, almost imperceptibly arching away from us post-Solstice, we sense that all our anticipation of summer has come to this—it's time to seize the day (and the night) and HAVE FUN. Virgo season will be here any moment, with its sharpened pencils and work ethic. But right now, in late July and the first three weeks of August, pleasure rules the roost. In the Northern Hemisphere, we are only a few months before the last harvest, and can pluck ripe fruit off trees or walk through tall fields of plants with a hot breeze blowing. We might grab cold cherries or plums from the fridge and let their sweetness run down our chin. In New York City, late summer heat and humidity are the great equalizer between the rich and poor that somehow bring all our bodies together in the shared bliss of an air-conditioned subway car after we almost melted on the platform. It's a very specific geographic summer joy, but trust me, it's pretty great.

Sex during Leo season can take on an athletic flair, spurred on by the energy we've been gifted by the extra vitamin D running through our veins. It's not just that people are outside wearing skimpy clothing that gets our engines running now (although this surely helps), but there is something about the middle of summer that can arouse us out of lethargy. When so much around us feels playful, it's hard not to want to get in the game, at least to throw one die. This season encourages frivolity, and knowing that the sex we can have doesn't need to be tied to heavy emotions might encourage us to experiment with a new partner.

Too much heat can be exhausting and we must stay hydrated, but in those first moments of the Sun hitting our face during Leo season mornings, we are often warmed up for that randy soul-to-sol connection.

## Get to Know the Sun, Leo's Ruling Luminary

Our survival on Earth depends upon the Sun—and so does our very existence. Billions of years from now, when the Sun burns out, all life on Earth will go with it. The Sun is our solar system's central star, and no wonder we worship it, from the Egyptian Ra to the Norse Sol to bikini-clad beachgoers trying to get that golden glow—it makes sense. We revolve around the Sun, and in turn, this ostentatious orb gives us limitless light.

The Sun is literally a life-giver—and astrologically, it helps us shine our own life-affirming light. Wherever the sun is, we can *see*. It is diurnal (of the daytime) and it illuminates everything it touches. It brings sharp clarity and allows us to witness what it reveals. In this way, it gives us a direction. I had a fair amount to say about the Sun in the introduction, so you may want to review those earlier sections.

## More on the Moon and Sun and Their Back-to-Back Seasons

The two summer signs aren't ruled by planets like the other ten signs. The Moon and the Sun are the cosmic bodies we're most familiar with in our everyday experiences on Earth, as they are both integral to our own planet's orbital path. We rise and sleep with them every night, encountering them in the skies above us as we go about our lives, whereas we often need a telescope to view the other planets, or at least have some rudimentary knowledge of sky surfing (astronomy) to do this with the naked eye.

The Moon is of the emotional body while the Sun is of the soul and what it projects outward. The Moon corresponds to the unconscious and things that are buried, hidden, and private, while the Sun in our charts corresponds to consciousness, ego, and public acclaim—the things we do and feel that are visible to us and others.

As we move from our Moon season (Cancer) to our Sun season (Leo), we can flow from an inward gaze to an outward gaze, interior to exterior. Somewhat counter-intuitively, many people find it easier to feel into their natal chart's Moon, indicative of their inner terrain, than their Sun, which is what they exude. That may be because we're intimately involved with what is inside of us—our constantly shifting emotional needs— than we are with what we are radiating outward.

The Sun emits while the Moon receives. No matter where our natal chart's Moon sign is, we can use these two consecutive seasons of the luminaries to better understand the parts of our erotic selves that feel private—just for us—versus the parts that we want to show off and share with lovers, if that's our intention.

## Leo's Erotic Gifts

There's a reason sex parties are often called "play parties"—because when sex is the most pleasurable and free, we're in a state of creative, generative play. And that is the central erotic gift of Leo—the ability to tap into the restorative energy of erotic play. When they're at their best, Leos can tap this space unencumbered by heavy emotions or attachments. This is not to say they don't love deeply; rather, they convey that they know how to bring a sense of play to sex, even when their feelings are powerful. Whether they're enjoying solo sex or radiating their light to a partner, FUN is often the operative word.

As a fixed fire sign, Leos can create a container of erotic pleasure that keeps them not just warm but at exactly the right temperature. All the world is a stage, and for Leos, the bedroom is sometimes the best setting in which to tap into their purest creative instincts and come alive. When they're totally tapped into this instinct, they are genuinely sexually generous. There is a sense of optimism and belief that pleasure is an infinite well from which they can forever draw and share. There is a lavishness to the way that they love that can inspire their lovers, even lovers who lack the kind of natural confidence that a solar-charged Leo often possesses.

Leo's other erotic gift is vitality—an aliveness and passion for living life fully and robustly and refusing to waste it. For all the fire signs, there can be a sense that their entire being wakes up when they are aroused, and with Leos, this can come across as a contagious joy.

The first time I had sex with a Leo man, it was someone I'd met in a bar an hour earlier. Something about him made me, an unusually shy Aries, march right up to him, extend my hand, and say, "Hi, I'm Stefanie, who are you?" Within ten minutes we were making out, and suddenly I was back at his place. I later realized how inspired I was by his easy confidence, and even though I had no idea who he was, even from across the room, he radiated a mesmerizing glow that drew me over.

There was a problem, though—at least for how I imagined having a first sexual encounter with someone: I had my period! Period sex is something I'm all for, but for me, not necessarily the first time. I didn't expect to sleep with him, but his oozing charisma put me in a state of "Well, let's just go and see what happens." I told him I had my period, and he was totally unflummoxed. He tore off my panties, ripped out my tampon, and we proceeded to have the most athletic, playful, fun sex I'd had in a long time.

This man, who was a multi-hyphenate creative—a painter, actor, and yoga instructor—radiated his Leonian light so brightly that it created a vortex that pulled me in. But Leo's many erotic gifts are not about the suction of seduction that their energy can create across an expanse—it's about how they fuel themselves with this fire, generating a creative loop that feels like it's powered by a Sun that will never burn out. Some Leos, like my tampon-tugging friend, can keep up this energy all night (or day), and it can be exhausting for their lovers. Leo's primary erotic gift is their vitality and playfulness—the dazzling confidence just helps them get what they want.

## Pathway to Play and Creativity for Leo

No matter a Leo's actual profession, they are often artists of some sort. Painters, actors, musicians, writers, sculptors, designers, dancers—you'll find tons of Leos among them. But even the buttoned-up business types might secretly long to make a creative splash. If there is any sign at all who NEEDS to express and emote through art, it's Leo. When a Leo is depressed or anxious, sexually frustrated or insecure, finding a creative outlet is the healthiest way for them to heal. This functions as a container for what their wild heart feels, allowing them to return to a state of openness and play.

## Leo's Erotic Challenges

The need for outsized attention can stymie a Leo's erotic flow and create roadblocks to pleasure. Leos can sometimes get away with faking it 'til they make it, but that can only take them so far, and it only works when they really believe in their mission. If something has burned up their confidence, especially their sexual confidence, they can fall into the trap of not being able "to perform"—this might mean losing erections or experiencing vaginismus or just plain low libido, so they're not inspired to have sex, even with themselves.

For Leos, even one bout of performance anxiety can feel like forgetting their lines once the curtain rises, and it can cause deep humiliation. They must learn that not everyone can be "on" all the time, and that they're not disappointing or failing themselves (or a lover) if they don't feel like showing up for sex now and again.

If a Leo's creativity is blocked in their work or daily life, it can spread to their sex life suddenly and unexpectedly. Like the Sun quickly darting behind the clouds, Leos are often surprised and shocked that their innate vitality isn't there when they want to access it. Looking to whether they genuinely have a creative outlet is a wise first step. A Leo must have a place to experiment, play, and perform, or else they can feel like they're dying on the vine.

When a Leo finds themselves being sexually *performative* rather than *genuinely creative*, they can lose their mojo. Think of the way that women moan and scream in stereotypical porn, the kind made for cishet men. When a Leo keeps going more and more over the top to convince themselves (or their lovers) that everyone is having fun, even when they're not, or to comfort a lover into believing they're desirable or sexually skilled—that's performative pleasure. When a Leo slips into bad acting or overcompensation, it can feel to them like they've flubbed their lines so badly that they never want to return to the stage, and a self-created humiliation spiral might ensue.

Leos prefer to put everything they've got on the page or the stage, so any sense that they have to keep their sexual "failures" to themselves—to store them as some kind of shameful secret—can just make the situation worse. Once a Leo becomes self-conscious, they can stop radiating their glow, and once the glow is muted, sometimes the only thing that can bring it back is applause. So once the Leo disappoints themselves, they may seek validation from others and fall into a "Who is the most beautiful (sexy, sexually skilled, orgasmic, the best lover ever, insert your over-the-top compliment here) of them all?" phase that echoes loudly over and over. When that swagger stops, even if friends and lovers don't realize it's gone, the Leo can deflate and turn in on themself—and that is how they might lose touch with their erotic drive.

## Leo Shame and Shadow Work

Leo's opposite sign is Aquarius, best known for its cool, calm, collected detachment and superior analytical skills. Leo energy can feel like it's all heart, all the time. Their shadow is a sign often accused of being detached and emotionless (although it's a lot more complicated than that).

Leos must remember not to take up every ounce of oxygen in a room, simply because they're so keen to be seen. Their Aquarius shadow can show them that their need to be acknowledged is likely not as dramatic as they feel like it is in the moment.

When a Leo struts so wildly that they take up all the attention in a showy way, instead of just letting their natural glow do the work, it may be because deep inside, they fear not feeling anything at all. This is a royal sign that's well known for loyalty, and it's often said that Leos will kill for their beloveds—but all that drama just might be overcompensation.

It is widely believed that one of the most infamous Leos in history, Napoleon, launched a war and ended up imprisoned to make up for his supposed lack of height (turns out this was a myth perpetuated by the British). There is nothing wrong with being short or having a body that in any way doesn't comport with societal standards for beauty and attractiveness—this goes without saying. But the "Napoleon Complex" refers to the way shorter men sometimes engage in toxic masculinity (like starting wars) in order to show everyone how lovable they are. When it comes down to it, all a Leo wants is to be loved and told that they're loved, early and often. All hail short kings, but this guy clearly illustrates the trap Leos can fall into when their self-confidence is weakened.

It's normal for all human bodies to slow down with age, and it's normal for even young bodies to get tired now and then. And it's also normal and common for people to be born into bodies that have or develop chronic illnesses, or have accidents, and so on—all common life experiences that can change sexual functioning. Yet when Leos experience a body or energy level that is different than they expect, they might take it personally—even more so than people of other signs.

Janine was a transwoman, pansexual performance artist, and pole dancer in her midthirties when she was referred to me by another client. After suffering a debilitating back injury and having to pull back from her work life for six months, she began feeling despondent and her libido precipitously dropped. She had four regular partners, including one live-in lover, but two months into her recovery, she felt compelled to end these relationships entirely. The only one that remained in her life was her live-in partner, as he couldn't afford to move out.

She told me: "I feel like my body will never work again, and that makes me feel undesirable." We looked at the ways she learned, both in childhood and later in her teens and twenties, to always be "on" in order to feel loved, especially in the years before she came out as trans. We then began to unpack all the ways that her body was, indeed, not merely desirable but capable of experiencing desire, and that slowing down temporarily was not the same thing as being imprisoned alone on an island. We talked about small, less athletic, safe ways she could continue to pleasure herself, and she invested in hands-free sex toys designed for people with accessibility issues, and they were a big hit. Eventually, she felt brave enough to invite her lovers back to be intimate with her again, and their relationships deepened and grew.

When a body changes and can't move as quickly, lithely, or athletically as it did in its prime, the frustration can mount and create a kind of sexual shutdown. Finding new, creative ways to engage erotically is key, before too much time passes and they begin to see themselves as people who used to enjoy eroticism, but fear they never will again. To a certain extent, all the fire signs have a very hard time with aging and their changing bodies, but Leo's fixed quality can make them feel like all emotions and identities are permanent, especially the uncomfortable ones.

In partnerships, it's important for a Leo to communicate that they require regular praise. One way of doing this is offering compliments to a lover, and hoping they do the same in return. But another is saying, "I love it when you tell me how hot I am during sex." Praise play comes out of the BDSM scene and it's perfect for Leos and their lovers. Simplified, it's just the act of telling your partner how amazing they are before, during, or after sex.

A Leo who has done their shadow work is in confident command of their sexuality, having and often providing a very good time. Committed sex, robust and fiery sex, casual sex, athletic sex, or slow and sensual sex to accommodate a changing body—whatever kind of sex a Leo chooses to have, they choose their pleasure with their full attention and little second-guessing.

## Journal Questions for Leo Shadow Work

- What do I radiate erotically?
- How would I feel if the applause stopped?
- How am I proud of myself?
- Would I love myself if I slowed down?
- I deserve to play, no matter what my body looks like or feels like—how can I keep playing no matter what?
- If I tune into my heart, what does it tell me?

## A Deeper Look at Body Rulership and Erogenous Zones for Leo

Leo rules the most important organ, the heart—a body part that will instantly kill us if it stops beating for too long. Just like the Earth can't function without the Sun, Leo's ruling luminary, the heart, is central to all emotional and sexual functioning in the Leo body. For Leos, the inner Sun is their heart, and they must walk the Earth guided by its dictates.

A basic Leo tenet is that everything must be heart-centered, which is not to say overly dramatic, emotional, or self-serious. But even in the most casual, non-committal romantic or sexual situations, their heart must be in it for it to feel good. Feeling authentic love for oneself and one's lover(s) will keep that heart energy radiating brightly and can keep a Leo in a state of play rather than a state of performance.

Taking good care of the heart in the way that cardiologists recommend is a no-brainer—but paying close attention to the heart chakra and listening to its energetic messages is also necessary. The heart, as an organ, is in the same area as the heart chakra, an energetic center of the body that is thought to govern love and self-love (see illustration on page 19). Checking in with the heart might mean doing heart chakra opening yoga poses like Cobra Pose (lie flat on your stomach, place your hands underneath your shoulders, inhale, and gently push up until your back is slightly arched, then return to a flat position), heart chakra meditations (easily found online), or just bringing hands to heart occasionally throughout the day to tune in with its beating.

During solo or partnered sex, taking a deep breath and listening to one's own heartbeat or a lover's can deepen the connection markedly, heightening pleasure. Some options for heart-centered erotic play: putting one's head to a lover's chest to listen to their heart, laying a hand on their heart, or listening simultaneously to both hearts, with one hand on one's own chest and the other on a lover's.

Leo also rules the thoracic spine and back, and all varieties of back massage can be tremendous turn-ons if available. From light touch to deep tissue, including back scratching and tracing fingers along the spine, this is where cat people excel—both as givers and receivers. Having back scratchers, electronic massagers, or a foam roller on hand can be super helpful for the Leo who wants to attend to their back. The human Leo body often feels instinctively feline and wants to experience movement and pleasure like a cat does. This can include something as simple as languid stretches, but in the act of sex, might mean lots of stroking—and not just of the genitals.

## An Embodiment Exercise for Leo Season

### Staring Into the Erotic Self

This powerful exercise can be emotionally confronting, depending on where you are on your healing path, so give yourself time and space afterward to sit quietly and process what you've experienced. This exercise requires privacy, a full-length mirror, and hopefully a door that locks so you won't be intruded on.

I often tell clients to perform this exercise in the nude, but if it feels too triggering, consider remaining clothed and beginning slowly by just focusing on the head, face, and upper body, and then coming out of the exercise. Stand in front of a mirror, looking at your face. Locking eyes with yourself, say these words: "You are beautiful, and I love you." Now begin looking closely at all your features, your hair, the shape of your face, your ears, neck, shoulders, chest/breasts, arms, fingers, belly, hips, pubic area, thighs, knees, calves, and finally your feet. As you scan each area, notice any criticism or cruelty that rises up, and replace it with "You are beautiful, and I love you." Now scan back up, lingering over any region that brought up difficult emotions or tension, and tell that part of your body "You are beautiful, and I love you." When you return to your face, look into your eyes one last time and say, "You are beautiful, and I love you." Now, put your hands on your heart, and say it one more time.

A person with low vision could do this exercise by moving their hands over their body as described above, feeling each body part and saying "I love you" as they go.

Remember, this exercise can be emotionally triggering. You may cry, laugh, feel silly, or find new parts of yourself to love. Consider writing in your journal about what you observed and how you felt.

## Try These Tools to Connect with Leo Energy:

- Experiment with praise play.

- Play naked twister or other childhood games with a lover.

- Try role-playing.

- Have sex at sunrise.

- Open your heart chakra.

- Take yourself on "artist dates"—a concept from Julia Cameron's wonderful book *The Artist's Way: A Spiritual Path to Higher Creativity.*

# 7

# Virgo Sexuality

## Perfection and Connection

There is no way to repress pleasure and expect
liberation, satisfaction, or joy.

**adrienne maree brown**

*Pleasure Activism*

**Dates:** August 21–September 21

**Sexual Archetype:** The Servant/Savior

**Motivation:** Efficiency

**Symbol:** The Virgin

**Planetary Ruler:** Mercury (also rules Gemini)

**Element:** Earth

**Modality:** Mutable

**Erogenous Zones and Body Rulership:**
The Abdomen, Digestive System, and
Sympathetic Nervous System

Healthy Virgo energy is attuned to nuance, attentive to detail, ripe
for personal transformation, delicate but grounded, practical,
smart as hell, efficient, a beacon of excellence, and a born hands-on

healer. Virgos often want to be *excellent* at everything, not merely competent, and sexual prowess is part of their repertoire of planned perfection. Yet when they feel overly responsible for every little thing, including their own pleasure and that of their partners, they can devolve into a loop of libido-killing anxiety and shame.

Many Virgos seem to have emerged from the womb with a sewing kit in their hand and toolbelt on their waist: they appear ready to fix everything, even things that don't seem broken. Yet when a Virgo has avoided doing their own shadow work, they're less equipped to fix their own personal mess(es). Privately, Virgos might feel overwhelmed by chaos, and by hypervigilantly correcting a partner's problems (or problems in their environment, like that toilet that needs scrubbing), they get to avoid doing their own agonizing inner work. When it comes to sexual relationships, this can be a source of conflict, because it takes two to make the thing go right.

Virgo is a deeply, deeply sensitive sign, but its sensitivity takes a different shape than that of Cancer, the cardinal water sign that we explored in chapter 5. As a mutable earth sign ruled by intellectual Mercury, Virgo tends to experience its sensitivity through a sharpness of mind rather than a suppleness of emotions. As an earth sign, Virgo speaks to a more material realm; its energy is often concretized, or at least made of soil to be shaped into something of substance.

### Hot for Teacher: Virgo Season in Focus

When Virgo season begins in late August—days might still be sticky but nights are getting slightly cooler in the Northern Hemisphere—we are reminded that most of the summer is in the rearview mirror already. The height of wild Leonian playtime has passed and we may start to think about heading back to school or work, depending on our personal circumstances. We might begin to feel nostalgia for a season that isn't even officially over, as we prepare to get down to the daily business of what comes next.

Even adults without children often have this seasonal pattern ingrained in their body-mind—the way late summer signals we're soon to head back to some kind of classroom. We are pruning and refining now. Maybe our summer Fridays off are about to evaporate after Labor Day, or our time at the lake or shore is soon to come to an end. The vibe is clear: shop for your clean notebooks and sharpen your pencils, because it's time to get organized. At the start of Virgo season, the seasonal hinge of the autumnal equinox is still a month away, but we become more aware of the calendar now. In the bright heat of midsummer, days may have melted into one another, seemingly without end. If we stopped popping meetings into our schedule during early summer vacation, or began leaving work early, or took a few extra-long weekends, we might realize that those blocks are starting to fill up again. This is but one of the ways that Virgo season modulates the excesses of Leo season.

We also might find ourselves thinking about the abundant health benefits of sex, rather than focusing on wild romance. We are moving back inward now, less concerned about impressing lovers with big-hearted gestures or athletic sexual positions, and perhaps more worried that we took one of our summer sex dramas a little too far. We might make to-do lists about sexual health, refill our spent bottles of lube with organic varieties, invest in new bed linens, and book a pelvic floor therapy session just to make sure sexual wellness is part of our overall health routine.

In Virgo season, some of us might admonish ourselves for having been a touch too lazy, having had too much fun, or overindulging in summer play when we believe we should be serious grownups. Some of us might get super excited about our next trip to the Container Store. Virgo season can motivate us to launch self-improvement projects, from home office reorganization to juice cleanses to creating ambitious fall reading lists.

There is still abundant light, but it is softening, becoming less aggressive and crisp, and even though peak foliage won't happen until later, we might sense that the leaves are preparing to transition to their next phase. Virgo season brings to mind rows of fields waiting to be harvested later in the fall, and the final touches of cultivation they require. Our days might have more complexity as we assimilate our long, lazy summer into our busy fall schedules. By mid-Virgo season, around September 5, this all usually begins to make sense.

Like a Virgo body, associated with the abdomen, we are focused on digesting the end of the summer season and preparing to give it a new form: the fall. Our sympathetic nervous systems (the part of the nervous system that controls our "fight-or-flight" mechanism) might be more active now as we adapt new details and duties. If we don't find healthy outlets to process the stress of increased workloads, we can feel frazzled. At the same time, like over-eager teacher's pets, we might sit at the front of the class ready to absorb Virgo season's detailed lessons with our hands raised.

## Get to Know Mercury, Virgo's Planetary Ruler (Again)

Mercury, the messenger planet, also rules the sign of Gemini. (You can flip back to chapter 4 to read more about the myth and history of this fascinating nonbinary deity associated with the Greek god Hermes.) The intellectual energy and frenetic drive are similar in each sign, but because Virgo is a mutable earth sign, its denizens can find ways to channel their brainpower into a singular task and stick with it until it's completed, unlike Gems, who tend to get bored quickly unless the subject changes every few minutes. This mutability can make Virgos into little Energizer Bunnies that thrive when busy fixing things (and people) rather than communicating about it like airy Geminis.

The way that each sign experiences their relationship with their planetary ruler is different. Mercury is exalted in Virgo, but not in Gemini; this is just a way of saying Mercury is more comfortable and at home in Virgo. The shared essence is movement: Mercury in both signs must constantly move, and, like Hermes on the road, it's about the journey, not the destination, although Virgo revels in the sense of completion of a task well accomplished.

## Virgo's Erotic Gifts

Virgo sexuality has nothing to do with prudery. Because the Virgo symbol is the Virgin, some people mistakenly assume Virgos represent puritanism or display a moralist disinterest in sex and pleasure. Our culture's mixed-up messages about virginity and "purity culture" contribute to this confusion. Many Virgos connect deeply with the idea that they are complete unto themselves—a Virgo archetype. A major erotic asset of Virgo is their affinity for going solo and feeling fine about it.

Virgo is associated with The Hermit card of the Tarot, a symbol of clarity, the kind that is achieved without distraction or contagion. There are Tarot card associations for every sign and not all are included in this book, but I'm sharing this one because it shows us a striking truth about the Virgo temperament. The Hermit understands that they must sometimes sequester themselves far away from other humans in order to connect to the purity of unadulterated wisdom. Virgos, when healthy and aligned, can experience erotic clarity—they know exactly what their body wants and how to get it. And while erotic clarity means many different things to many different people, healing and reconnecting to the body—behind the noise of the mind—is a major part of the sexual journey for Virgos.

Scholars of astrology believe the virgin/maiden associated with Virgo's astrological glyph represented the temple priestess or sacred prostitute in Sumer and Babylonia, which is to say, the one married to the deity. These priestesses often lived at the temple and had sex with men who would come to honor the goddess. In this way, they were unavailable for marriage, and wholly self-possessed. Like these priestesses, when a Virgo's nervous system is calm and they are clear on their desires, they can stand apart from others, without needing external validation, confident in their erotic value and their body's ability to experience pleasure that is both spiritual and health-giving.

As the lightest of the earth signs, a Virgo's agility is one of their top erotic assets. Grounded in the principles of sex as a healing modality, the therapeutic principle of "a little goes a long way" can encourage them to use pleasure as medicine on a daily basis. This is a sign that's often willing to try different healing modalities to reduce stress, from homeopathy to yoga to having an orgasm a day to keep the doctor away. Their exquisite attention to detail is often a huge sexual asset. Whether this helps them to direct a lover to the right spot on their body or encourages them to ask a partner questions and experiment with different kinds of touch until they get it right—sexual perfection is something they may strive for, to everyone's benefit.

This means that Virgos should attend to their gut feelings so they can experience regular, sustained, health-giving pleasure on a daily basis. They might be one of the signs best equipped to thrive with regular "sex dates" whether they're with a partner or having solo sex. "Why not put a masturbation sesh in my calendar?" a Virgo might say.

Sexual healing is Virgo's birthright and mission. They are both the alchemists and purifiers of the cosmos. They are driven to identify separate pieces and bits, and then meld them all together as a satisfied whole. For an integrated, healthy Virgo, the pleasure is in the details.

## Pathway to Play and Creativity for Virgo

Virgos endure a stereotype that says they're uptight and boring, thus less creative, which I'll happily call bullshit on right now. As one of the quickest studies of the zodiac, Virgo can throw itself at almost any creative endeavor, then focus and finish with aplomb. With their exquisite organizational skills, all kinds of handicrafts may call to them, especially anything that weaves a pattern and has repetitive steps, like knitting or quilting. Note that not all Virgos are neat! Some of them live in a state of barely controlled chaos, but there is still a perfectionist in there someplace. Often, the messiest Virgos are going through a tough time and feeling anguished, and the slightly messy Virgos have had a breakthrough and know they can still feel safe even when a few things are out of place. Their nervous systems are soothed when they keep their hands busy and there are steps to follow. Completely letting go of an end result may be hard but deeply rewarding for Virgos, so playing with colored sand sculptures or other ephemeral artworks might intrigue.

In the erotic realm, Shibari (Japanese rope bondage) can be incredibly fun, stress relieving, and hot.

## Virgo's Erotic Challenges

Criticism, rigidity, and a tendency toward fight-or-flight reactions can take a Virgo out of the pleasure game before they've even laid a card down on the table. Virgos may feel like they have to do everything right before they can show up for satisfying sex. This might mean being perfectly plucked or buff, being dressed right, studying kissing techniques, and that thing next to godliness: being perfectly clean. A stray hair missed by the waxer can throw some of them into a spiral of worry, killing off the potential for pleasure. A dirty sheet can do this, too. Even for solo sex, certain Virgos may be instantly turned off by anything that feels unclean or less than eat-off-the-floor hygienic.

They can turn this criticism on themselves, which is common, but also on their lovers, falling into that classic unhealthy relationship habit: trying to fix their partner. Understandably, sexual performance critiques are not always relished, and being nagged about the way one left the toothpaste uncapped can grow tiresome. When Virgos are disappointed in themselves, stressed, or experiencing a dysregulated nervous system, they can project a need for efficiency—getting straight to the point. This might mean sex without foreplay, or something that helps them (or their partner) achieve a quick orgasm, just to get it done. Not that there's anything wrong with that! But if all sexual activity is merely efficient and lacks soul, emotional connection, or layers of pleasure, it can end up making a Virgo or their partner feel like the spark is gone. Often, when a Virgo feels compelled to criticize their partner, a delicate and intricate dance is going on in their own psyche. If we drilled down deep enough, we might find the Virgo struggling with intrusive thoughts and their own inner critic, unable to forgive themselves for failing to be perfect at something. Facing that sometimes-vicious inner critic, one that's likely plagued them since childhood, can be something they'll try to avoid at all costs, even if that means antagonizing someone they truly love and are attracted to.

The fear of letting go and losing control can keep a Virgo from experiencing nearly spiritual levels of pleasure that are possible for them. At the core, many Virgos just want to be of service, but unhealthy levels of obsessive/compulsive perfectionism can end up costing them access to the healthy, robust sexuality that should be their birthright.

## Virgo Shame and Shadow Work

A Virgo's fear of inner chaos comes in part from their opposite sign and shadow—Pisces. This is the last sign of the zodiac, where the end is the beginning, and all energy and matter flow together in their infinite sea. Messy Virgos and perfectionist Virgos both struggle with integrating their fear of chaos.

Virgo's addiction to order and perfection is in stark contrast to the hot, beautiful mess of their Pisces shadow. This is a sexual and spiritual predicament, especially if Virgo is unwilling to get over their constant criticism and go with the erotic flow.

A queer cis male Virgo client of mine was in a long-term committed relationship with his partner, and they were struggling to connect with each other sexually after seven years of maintaining a hot erotic bond. Joseph's partner David (an Aries) wanted to open the relationship—but this was a no-go for Joseph. Joseph was still wildly attracted to his partner, but because of work stress, he felt irritable and knew he was taking it out on David. He began to complain about the way David cleaned the kitchen after cooking, creating domestic tensions that they'd happily avoided until now.

Joseph was also losing a battle with his libido. He wanted to connect sexually with his beloved but began experiencing erectile issues, and yet pushed himself to make sure David got at least three flawless blowjobs a week—he felt that he would lose him if he didn't perform this as a duty. Even though he felt compelled to be of service sexually because they had an early agreement to be GGG (good, giving, and game), he began feeling resentful about it. David would offer to reciprocate, but Joseph would turn over and go to sleep. He also entirely stopped masturbating around this time.

It's natural for people in relationships to experience differences in libido at various times in their partnership, and it's common for men in their forties (Joseph was forty-six when I met him) to experience a decrease in testosterone that softens their libido. But Joseph, struggling with his need to be perfect—the perfect lover, the perfect employee, the perfect infallible human—was at first unreceptive to this information. He wanted a solution to fix it, so I suggested erectile medication. At first, he said no. As a long-time yogi, vegan, and eschewer of pharmaceuticals, it felt antithetical to his entire ethos.

Before calling me, he'd spent hours on the internet searching for what might be wrong with him, going down many rabbit holes and considering all kinds of supplements, penis pumps, and other erectile dysfunction paraphernalia.

Eventually he agreed to try Cialis, and at first, this worked well, because it solved the problem, making Joseph feel virile again and helping David to feel desired so that he stopped asking to open the relationship. Yet after a few months, Joseph came in for a session feeling depressed and unsatisfied. He complained that their entire sex life felt like just another job for him, a place where he had to show up and serve. He revealed that he had a pattern of getting into this kind of less-than-reciprocal relationship, where he eventually felt like the only one who was giving anything, sexually and otherwise.

We began to dig deeper into why Joseph felt compelled to fix his relationships without asking his partners to do any real work. It was almost as if he set up scenarios where he could never not be in control, and we discovered that it stemmed from a messy, toxic childhood, where his alcoholic mother constantly overslept and left young Joseph to fend for himself in the mornings, cleaning up the dinner dishes, making himself breakfast, and getting himself to the school bus. Joseph tried desperately to cling to control as an adult to ensure he never ended up in a situation like his chaotic childhood again.

This is a fairly common dysfunctional Virgo scenario: they end up becoming rigid and controlling in their relationships as a way of avoiding the chaos that they feel inside. For vulva-havers, this can present as vaginismus and anorgasmia. It's hard for libido to flow under these conditions, no matter how many different modalities they try to "fix" it. Often relief comes in the form of exhaling and letting go. Sometimes, if the Virgo is forced to give up control of a situation with great anguish, they realize afterward that they could have chosen to surrender instead. Either way, they often find that everything hasn't fallen apart, and hopefully take that lesson with them into their next experience.

As Joseph unpacked the very old trauma that he'd locked inside of him for many decades, he also, at my urging, began attending EMDR sessions and received bodywork. After a few months, his stress levels plummeted and he felt like himself again, with his nervous system now regulated. He then realized that HE wanted to open up the relationship! Being back in touch with his gut instinct made Joseph realize he wanted to experience more sexual experimentation. Several years later, Joseph and his partner are still together and continue to thrive in their consensual non-monogamous partnership.

The way into Virgo shadow work can sound simple but feel difficult, and yet it's essential for Virgo well-being, both in bed and out. They need to stop projecting their own self-criticism onto the people they love and desire. Turning off their own internal critic can turn their sexuality back on.

## Journal Questions for Virgo Shadow Work

- What does the word "chaos" evoke for me?
- What would happen if I completely relaxed during sex?
- How much can I write about a lover or past lover before I want to criticize them?
- Where is that criticism coming from?
- What would happen if I talked back?
- What would happen if I lost control?

## A Deeper Look at Body Rulership and Erogenous Zones for Virgo

Because Virgo's body rulership doesn't offer us a specific body part to explore other than the abdomen, one of the best ways to play with their erogenous zones is to stimulate and calm the nervous system.

The vagus nerve is the longest nerve in our bodies. It is a cranial nerve leading from the top of the spine to the stomach—traversing the entire brain-gut axis as part of the parasympathetic nervous system. It wraps around the neck and connects to the heart as well. It relates to the "rest and digest" function of our bodies and is responsible for digestion, cardiovascular functions, heart rate, breathing, and reflexes. In short, when it is dysregulated, our anxiety can skyrocket. Paying attention to the regulation of the vagus nerve can be incredibly beneficial for soothing high-strung Virgo nervous systems, providing grounding and bringing calm, and in turn, improving their relationship to their sexual selves. Self-regulation through vagus nerve stimulation might look like:

- Gentle massage behind the ear or tugging on the ear

- Gentle and careful massage of the side of the neck where your carotid artery pulse is felt

- Gargling, humming, and singing

- Immersing your face in very cold water

- Lying on your right side

- The 4-7-8 breathing method (inhale for four seconds through the nose, gently hold the breath for seven seconds, and then exhale for eight seconds)

Syncing breath up with a lover is a wonderful practice for co-regulation of the nervous system. This is sometimes called circular breathing. It's pretty simple and can be done before sex, during sex, after sex, or just sitting at the breakfast table. You can do this lying down, sitting up, or standing. Facing one another, put your hand on their heart, chest, or belly. Just holding hands can enhance the practice, as can doing it naked. Begin by taking three deep breaths together, then listen closely, trying to softly attune to your partner's breath. Stay synced for a while, then pause after an exhale, waiting for them to inhale so you're making a circle. Keep going like this as long as it feels good.

## An Embodiment Exercise for Virgo Season

### Being of Service to Yourself

Try to clear a space in your schedule when you can be completely alone for at least a half hour—ideally an hour. If you live with other people, try to do this when everyone else is out, but a locked bedroom door is a solid second choice. If someone else is home, consider using white noise or music to mask sounds so you feel a sense of privacy. The only rule for this ritual is that you must not stop early to do something else. The purpose here is to let go of control in a space that is safe.

The light can be on or off, or you can use candlelight—whatever makes you feel safe in your body is best. Begin by closing your eyes if you feel comfortable and taking a breath deep into your belly, holding the breath for four counts, and then exhaling through your mouth or nose. Do this five more times or whatever feels right. Now open your eyes and remove as many of your clothes as you feel comfortable with—try for all of them!

Get into bed and close your eyes. Take five more deep belly breaths. Say out loud: "I am alone, and I am free. No one is judging me." Begin exploring your body with your hands, figuring out what feels good. Go slow. You may feel like this is silly or indulgent. You may start to feel turned on and want to immediately give yourself an orgasm, but refrain for now.

Thoughts like "This is ridiculous" or "I have to finish the laundry" could come up while you're doing this. When that happens, gently brush them away from the screen of your mind, take a few deep breaths, and come back to the sensation of exploring your body. Pay special attention to your neck and the area below your ears, using gentle or strong pressure—touch until you sense into what feels best.

Continue like this, returning to your breath and the quietness of your mind if intrusive thoughts or worries begin to emerge. After you've practiced this for at least a half hour, you can proceed to fantasizing, using a sex toy, or bringing yourself to orgasm using your hand—if you like. You certainly don't have to, but you may want to, so it's an option.

## Try These Tools to Connect with Virgo Energy:

- Soothe your nervous system with daily pleasure(s).
- Try a sensory-deprivation tank.
- Remember that self-care doesn't always require self-improvement.
- Don't clean up every mess.
- Make lists of your desires and turn-ons.

# 8

# Libra Sexuality

## Allure and Ambivalence

> Knowing how to be solitary is central to the art of
> loving. When we can be alone, we can be with others
> without using them as a means of escape.
>
> **bell hooks**
>
> *All About Love: New Visions*

**Dates:** September 21–October 21

**Sexual Archetype:** The Enchanter

**Motivation:** Partnership

**Symbol:** The Scales

**Planetary Ruler:** Venus (also rules Taurus)

**Element:** Air

**Modality:** Cardinal

**Erogenous Zones and Body Rulership:** The Kidneys,
Lumbar Region/Lower Back, and Endocrine System

Healthy Libra energy is poised, charismatic, charming, diplomatic, artistically sensitive, tranquil, reciprocal, relational, peaceful, and delightfully social. Yet Libras can lose focus and grow sexually unbalanced when they give their will away to their partners. Their secret is that even as very social animals, Libras don't necessarily want to be seen in a naked, genuine way. To maintain possession of their most potent sexual selves, they must find their inner fire and figure out how to be truly independent and authentic.

Light and dark. Yin and yang. Up and down. Back and forth. Libras often have trouble with one because it completely blots out the other until the pendulum swings back, revealing the polar opposite they've been missing. They may look perfectly put together and placid, conveying a calm exterior, but very often this flawless facade is a projection—the inner struggle for balance is real. Internally, Libras are constantly tossed and turned between potential outcomes and myriad choices. Because of this, they stereotypically hate having to make final decisions, from what to choose on a dinner menu to whom to commit to for life.

Libra's glyph is The Scales (they're the only sign not represented by a living being) indicating a sense of innate balance. Although Libras are known as justice seekers, diplomats, and peacemakers, if we dig deeper, we realize that all of these activities are built on offering peace to *other people*. But what about their own peace? True balance is their holy grail, their self-realization. They are on an eternal quest to find it, teetering from side to side of their scale depending on the situation or relationship they're in at any given moment.

## The Beautiful Ones: Libra Season in Focus

We meet Libra season at the hinge of the autumnal equinox in the Northern Hemisphere, when we must say a real goodbye to summer and find a way to make peace with the darkness that our bodies know is coming. Like the vernal equinox that introduced Aries season, the fall equinox brings us balance between light and dark—these are the only days of the year when there will be *equal* day and night in both hemispheres (the Southern Hemisphere begins their spring now). The elusive state of balance that Libras seek exists only at this moment, and natives of the sign often spend their entire lives trying to recreate it.

In Libra season days are shortening, leaves are starting to turn, and our circadian rhythms are pulsing with a new tempo. The march to deep fall (Scorpio season) intensifies as we move from the last days of September and further into October. The Virgoan state of clarity and purity we've just exited makes space for the company of other people, allowing us to reconsider the concept of "relationship." This is when singles begin to consider the merits of "cuffing season," waking up to colder days in which we might appreciate having someone already in the bed with us, rather than having to seek someone new. If we're going to be spending more time indoors, perhaps we don't want to do so alone.

As a bridge between Virgo season and Scorpio season, Libra season might feel like the sexual sweet spot between precision and urgency. Virgo often doles out its erotic energy furtively, overanalyzing every detail. Scorpio, the fixed water sign after Libra, can approach love and lust like a mysterious, heat-seeking missile that cannot be stopped until it gets what it obsessively wants. In Libra season, we may find ourselves wanting to create and be around beauty.

## Get to Know Venus, the Planetary Ruler of Libra (Again)

In Taurus, we encountered an earthy, grounded Venus (see chapter 3). In Libra, other qualities of Venus flourish.

Venus is the closest planet to Earth outside of our Moon and Mercury (depending on where it is orbiting). She reminds us that even though we are thousands of light-years away from other stars, we have a deep intimacy with our own solar system. We'll explore this in much more depth in the Venus chapter later in the book.

This stunning beauty of the cosmos has enchanted stargazers for millennia. Glamorous Venus creates a five-pointed star across our ecliptic as it orbits around the Sun every eight years. This is sometimes called the "five-petaled star," evoking a rose, the flower associated with this planet. Venus dazzles the eye as it appears as an evening star for half the year, warm and bright and inviting.

Venus has many moods, and Libras tend toward the fine art aspect of the planet. This is a sign generally more inclined to museum dates (unlike a Taurus, who might generally prefer naked gardening). As an intellectual air sign, Libra energy can feel a bit removed and at a distance, something/someone to admire but not necessarily to touch. Where a Venus-ruled Taurus might feel an erotic charge while rolling around in soil surrounded by wildflowers, a Venusian scene indeed, Libras often prefer not to get dirty; their erotic landscape is more aesthetically refined.

## Libra's Erotic Gifts

What does a Libra want? To create and be adjacent to beauty at all times—and that includes in a sexual context. Eroticism is high art for a Libra, and they're usually not short on creative ideas. When they get going on a sexy concept, they can create a magnum opus of erotic gorgeousness. This is sex that, if captured in a singular frame, could hang in a gallery: an elegant and alluring image where line, shape, space, value, form, texture, and color have all been considered. Libras tend to insatiably crave beauty. They often infuse an erotic artistry into their sexuality that other signs don't even think about, whether in partnered or solo sex. This includes a capacity for fantasy that is rather elaborate. The Libra fantasy life is often filmic— stories with iconic cinematography; a beginning, middle, and an end that provides catharsis and denouement, not just an orgasm.

But in real life, with partners, the Libra might wonder: Is the lighting right? Are the sheets high-thread count, sensually soft but not too slippery? Does the lamp on the night table function as a sought-after objet d'art? Even if a Libra ends up in a sexual situation that has been unplanned, say in the dark and somewhat scuzzy bathroom of a dive bar, they will somehow be able to make it beautiful; this is their gift. Their unconscious agenda? Serenity, the kind of exquisite experience that only full immersion in art can provide. Libras can paint a scene for sex that will live on like a still life long after the moment has passed. Partners often talk about specific sexual memories with their Libra lovers, ones that are indelibly marked in their minds, much like visiting an iconic museum and gazing at a famous painting.

Libras may not always feel balanced in their own body-mind as they sway on the seesaw of their justice-seeking souls, but they often make *other people* feel desired simply by being in their presence. Even for solo sex, this is a fundamental part of the Libran pleasure principle. The concept of give and take, of creating beauty and admiring it—it's a major part of Libra's erotic gift. Yet the performative instinct can triumph over the instinctual one—an idea we'll explore more in the next section.

Libras tend to focus on meeting a partner's erotic needs, rather than both sensing into and delivering it, as their Venusian sibling Taurus does. Although Libras may understand erotic dynamics almost automatically and can anticipate a lover's longings, when they channel that erotic generosity back to their own bodies, they activate a deeper, more meaningful kind of pleasure that they can come back to again and again.

When Libras are genuinely turned on, authentically in possession of their basest desires first, but including the full range of their sexual needs, they can engage their full breadth of erotic possibility, and there is nothing more beautiful to behold.

## Pathway to Play and Creativity for Libra

Libras very often find themselves living as artists, or at least art adjacent. Their inherent connection to beauty gives them an attraction to and affinity for fine art, design, fashion, interior decorating, architecture—anything that requires a refined eye for aesthetics. In some ways, they're always trying to make themselves into a walking, breathing, flawless masterpiece, and they can feel quite out of sorts if a brushstroke on that canvas of the self isn't quite right. Allowing themselves to just play, with no agenda, no idea of a magnum opus, no one to impress—letting themselves get dirty and feel their inner animal spirit in the act of creation—that's how creativity unlocks the erotic for Libra. Getting comfortable with making mistakes and experimenting with what feels "ugly" and socially unacceptable—that's how this sign balances their scales.

## Libra's Erotic Challenges

Companionship is often a Libran core craving, and because that's not something humans can control by their sheer will (although a Libra might try), this can end up being an erotic challenge. When a Libra senses that being exceedingly pliable and polite and catering to the whims of a partner is their ideal sexual role, they can forget their own pleasure entirely, just to make sure the companionship remains. Because for many Libras, the idea of being unpartnered can be very frightening. This fear can lead a challenging seesaw of passive-aggressive behavior and codependency.

Many Libras have a way of becoming invisible so they can't be scrutinized or seen. Sometimes this is an unconscious process, but often a Libra can intentionally and artfully construct a projection of beauty to mesmerize loved ones or new acquaintances into only seeing their pretty surface. Pisces, where Venus is exalted, also have this quality, although they tend to be less conscious of the projection.

A Libra can get stuck in that performative space where sensation is secondary to appearance, and they find themselves floating in the ether above their bodies to check on the aesthetic. Doormat syndrome is not uncommon for Libras of all genders. If a Libra aims to perform beauty for friends, family, neighbors, and strangers rather than examining their own desires, sexual satisfaction is likelier to be stymied. For a Libra to experience stimulating and expanding pleasure, they should stop thinking about how things *look* and open up to how they *feel* emotionally and physically, even when the sexual scene doesn't have flawless production values.

Libras can be impressively proficient at compartmentalizing. Even though Libra is a sign that professes to love being in relationship—a sign that loathes being alone and covets partnership almost at all costs—they can be rather secretly non-monogamous. They may even keep this longing as a secret from themselves, rather than hiding it from their partners as most people do when they stray. As we have discussed, consensual non-monogamy is a perfectly healthy, fair arrangement for many couples. But even though a Libra may crave sexual variety, they can be reluctant to broach this conversation and opt to cheat because of fear of conflict.

Even after a Libra has been married for twenty years, they might continue to weigh the pros and cons of committing. And the "bed death" that comes for many relationships at two or five or seven years may not faze a Libra. Because they're so good at controlling their own minds, they may not even feel like they're cheating while having a secret affair with an ex. Please note: people of all signs and charts can and do fail to keep up to their relational commitments. And for Libras, often the mind may wander but they won't allow their bodies to follow.

A Libra's compulsion to compromise can make it difficult to get into the darker, more mysterious, and potentially erotically promising elements of their romantic and sexual connections. Many Libras won't accept that at some point, every couple needs to have a first fight and occasionally argue to fully understand where the other is coming from. Some Libras despise and fear emotional conflict as if it's a dangerous virus. Quarreling can make them feel shaky and unwell.

It's not that Libras abhor arguments about ideas—many of them will engage in a spirited but friendly debate about politics, art, or social justice. It's just that when relationships are on the line, they'll often agree rather than fight for their point of view. Their topsy-turvy indecisiveness about mundane subjects can feel argumentative to their lovers, however, they're more than likely just simply (and compulsively) weighing all the options over and over.

Airy Libras can get stuck in their minds and lose their energetic connection with their own erogenous zones. This doesn't mean they'll necessarily waver in pleasuring a lover—it simply means that sometimes they may *perform pleasure* more than they experience it. Libras might sometimes, unfortunately, agree tó sexual liaisons they're not in the mood for as the consummate people-pleasers of the zodiac.

Completely losing oneself in the act of orgasm and showing one's "O-face" can feel like a risk to a Libra. In that moment, when they let go of control and give themselves over to pleasure, they are no longer painting, showing, or commissioning a still life—they are revealing their true self. A fear of being ugly can take over, and rather than allow themselves to lose control of the moment, they'll fake it, drawing pleasure from their lover's pleasure, rather than being swept away by their own.

## Libra Shame and Shadow Work

Libras can find themselves constantly chasing and/or avoiding their shadow by remaining in more superficial, socially acceptable romantic relationships. Their polarity with the hungry, horny-on-main opposite sign Aries can make them disdain anything that looks too animalistic, but they might be attracted to partners that are brash in bed. Before they've explored their own desire nature with the raw honesty this process deserves, the base erotic hunger that drives an Aries can make a Libra outwardly cringe. But if an aggressive, dominant lover is willing to keep up appearances in the world outside the bedroom, a Libra might be willing to partner with them.

Libras find their balance when they identify their real needs, stop being afraid to ask for what they want, and learn to act a little more assertive (like an Aries). Getting in touch with that fiery core, even if it scares them, can liberate them from societal conventions, especially being too nice, which often comes at their own expense. Once Libras learn to stand up for themselves and realize that sometimes, there *is* a right answer, not just a wishy-washy middle ground, they become all powerful—sexually and otherwise.

A cishet male client of mine (with five planets in Libra including his ascendant) told me that more than anything, he always wanted companionship and commitment with a lifelong partner with whom he could also have hot, passionate sex. This sounded like a textbook Libra wish list at first. Yet when I met him in his midforties, Tom admitted that he had cheated on all his long-term partners since his twenties, never quite landing on the fairy tale he imagined. His partners were attractive, successful, and in fields that allowed him to inhabit elite social circles in New York City. Notably, they came from different cultures and spoke a different native language than he did—which offered him a way of never being truly seen or known. Hiding behind a language barrier was just one way that he hid out within his relationships, avoiding a raw confrontation with intimacy and his sexuality by compartmentalizing his desires. Of course, one can fall in true and passionate love or deep friendship with anyone from any culture that is different than one's own or with those who speak different languages—but in our work together, we discovered that this was a telling pattern for Tom that went beyond his taste.

He never formed a deep, meaningful, satisfying sexual connection to these partners, even when he stayed with them for years. They were good companions and he genuinely cared for them like they were family—he just didn't deeply desire them from the start. Unlike in situations where desires fade over time and a spark can be lit again, when that desire never exists in the first place, it can be difficult to create it from scratch. For sexual connection and satisfaction, Tom had affairs with women he described as "sensually riveting."

He would come back to a few ex-lovers again and again, particularly one—an Aries that he'd dated years earlier and couldn't let go of. This woman was able to see his whole self, warts and all, and still wanted him—and it frightened him. Even twenty years after meeting, they had satisfying, hot and sweaty sex when they resumed their affair during the pandemic—the kind of sex he secretly craved as he navigated a long-term sexless relationship with his day-to-day partner.

Before reconnecting with his Aries ex, his sex drive had begun to wane, a combination of being on an SSRI and age-related testosterone decline. But this, of course, didn't have to mean the end of his sex life, because people over forty can continue to have robust and healthy sex lives. He assumed his current partner would reject the idea of opening their relationship, so he had never broached the subject. I introduced him to Janet W. Hardy and Dossie Easton's book *The Ethical Slut: A Practical Guide to Polyamory, Open Relationships, and Other Adventures* so he could better understand the workings of ethical, consensual non-monogamy, and after spending a few months weighing all his options, he asked his partner to read it too. Together, they decided that they would experiment with non-monogamous relationship models, and they're still together and trying it out.

With Libra, the craving for meaningfully deep erotic experiences can remain elusive until they let go of the idea of how things are supposed to look. Engaging in performative pleasure or choosing partners that satisfy more superficial values and relegating sexual satisfaction to the backburner can put out their spark. Libras find balance when they allow themselves to get dirty, to be socially unacceptable, and engage with their inner animal desire—knowing that this, too, can be beautiful.

## Journal Questions for Libra Shadow Work

- What makes me feel like an animal?
- What would happen if I wasn't beautiful?
- What if my lover left me?
- What would it mean to be alone?
- If everything were stripped away from me and no one could look at me, what would I really, truly desire?

## A Deeper Look at Body Rulership and Erogenous Zones for Libra

Libra rules the lower back, where so much of our body's tension is stored. If left unaddressed, stress and back pain can cause myriad health issues for all, but especially Libras. Taking special care to gently stroke, caress, and nurture this part of the Libra body is essential. Having a supportive desk chair, a lumbar pillow in the car, and/or a knee pillow for sleeping that supports the spine are wise choices. Investing in regular massage with a gifted practitioner is highly recommended. If back issues haven't come up yet it may not seem urgent to tend to this part of the body, but for people with Libra planets, this TLC can never happen too early.

In partnered and solo sex for Libra, gentle massage of the lower back, light scratching, and supporting the low back can feel intensely pleasurable. Using pillows to support the back during sex, or experimenting with sex pillows or chairs can markedly increase Libran pleasure.

Libras tend to have sensitive kidneys and must stay hydrated, before, during, and after sex, and they should always be conscious about urinating after sex to avoid UTIs. (Everyone should do this! But especially Libras.) Libra also has rulership over the endocrine system and can be hormonally sensitive, and sometimes prone to blood sugar issues.

## An Embodiment Exercise
## for Libra Season

### Orgasm like an Animal

All signs can balance their shadow by experimenting with their opposite signs' traits and tendencies, but this is especially crucial for the Libra. Drawing out Aries-style animal passion, the kind that may look less than aesthetically pleasing, can be challenging for them, but oh so worth it. If a Libra wants to begin to find or relocate a lost sexual appetite, they must fire up a passion that is *theirs and theirs alone*, not shaped by or attuned to a partner's tastes (past or present). If they eschew, at least for a moment, the ways societal standards have shaped their relationship with their own body, it can unlock a hunger they may not have previously known. Sex with or in bodies that don't meet societally acceptable standards can be just as good as sex in bodies that look like whatever "beautiful" means to an individual Libra.

This is a very simple practice that doesn't call for anything elaborate, but privacy is essential, because it can get loud. If you live with others, you may want to have music on, or a loud television, just as long as the sounds aren't too distracting. If you usually use a sex toy to masturbate, or your hand and some lube, have those available.

If you're accustomed to fantasizing to turn yourself on, feel free to engage that part of your mind before you touch yourself. You can also watch porn—do whatever you want, as long as bringing yourself to orgasm feels possible. Your only mission is to tap into your inner animal, even if (and especially if) it feels aggressive or primal.

Ask yourself: Do you usually moan loudly during partnered sex, if you're having it? If the answer is yes, here is a second question: Are these sounds for you or for your lover? If you answered your lover, during this practice, you will let yourself get loud *only for your own pleasure.* As you get closer to orgasm, increase the volume. Notice whether you're judging the sounds you're making as too feral or loud. Keep going, and try grunting even if you usually make only polite, soft moans or stay entirely silent.

As you get closer to orgasm, keep getting louder, and then as you release into a paroxysm of pleasure, let go of any pretense and just be where you are. This may feel weird or performative at first, but think of it like taking a boxing class instead of a yoga class—it's exercising a series of muscles that you already possess, just in a new way. It doesn't mean you have to do it like this every time—it just means you are capable of it.

Additional option: if you have an easy way to record yourself using your phone, consider setting up a tripod so it records just your face. Watch the recording and pay special attention to your face during orgasm. Find the beauty in this, even if you want to judge it. Keep watching it until you stop judging it.

## Try These Tools to Connect with Libra Energy:

- Keep your environment aesthetically pleasing, whatever that means to you—especially when sex is on the menu. (Don't let anyone tell you you're being high-maintenance.)

- Alternatively, experiment with scenes that feel raunchy or dirty, whatever that means to you, and see what kind of erotic feelings come up.

- In social situations, experiment with making yourself the main character, taking up all the space in the room, and being first to talk rather than being polite.

- When you have the choice between spending time alone or with someone you aren't over the moon for, opt to go solo, just to see how you feel.

- Tap into any repressed rage and let it out in a physical way. You might try shaking it out, if that feels comfortable to you, yelling into a pillow, or even take an intense dance or kickboxing class.

# 9

# Scorpio Sexuality

## Metamorphosis and Magic

I desire the things which will destroy me in the end.

**Sylvia Plath**

*The Unabridged Journals of Sylvia Plath*

**Dates:** October 21–November 21

**Sexual Archetype:** The Sorcerer/Sorceress/Sorcerex

**Motivation:** Regeneration

**Symbol:** The Scorpion

**Planetary Ruler:** Mars (Traditional, also rules Aries)
and Pluto (Modern)

**Element:** Water

**Modality:** Fixed

**Erogenous Zones and Body Rulership:**
The Reproductive System, Genitals, Bowels,
and Excretory System

**H**ealthy Scorpio energy is impassioned, piercing, penetrating, powerful, psychologically astute, emotionally vulnerable (but secure), intense, intriguing, undeniably magnetic, and potent in presence.

Scorpio can take on investigations of intimate matters like no other sign, navigating the deep roots of sex, love, and desire.

Scorpio's emotional vulnerability is both their greatest asset and their biggest foil—adjusting to the intense volume of their feelings can take a lifetime of practice. If they try to control outcomes too tightly to avoid being hurt, a Scorpio can close themselves off from the ecstatic sexual experiences they could otherwise use as regenerative fuel.

Scorpios seem to have a way of stripping things down to the bare essentials of survival, throwing everything else in life into stark relief. The absolute fragility of human experience can become clear in the presence of Scorpio energy, a sense that death could come at any moment, so why not live this one life with the intensity of a thousand splitting atoms?

I liken Scorpios to human microscopes that have the power to make anyone under their gaze feel like a biological sample they're carefully probing for clues. Scorpios often know how to construct an accurate map of the human psyche, which they might carefully plot out, starting by observing the subject with their penetrating stare. When Scorpios do this, it's generally because this fixed water sign likes to be in control of energetic and emotional exchanges, just in case they need to wield that power later on. This is a strategy of self-protection.

Scorpios don't often express outward, visible panic. Their fixed water energy rarely seems to fully boil over the edge of their cauldron, remaining on simmer for as long as is needed to keep everyone within their circle of trust safe and warm. It's no wonder that triple Scorpio Björk wrote a song in which she says that a "state of emergency" is "so beautiful" to her. Scorpios can dive hungrily into what other signs might see as dangerous extremes, or just hang out close to the edge, quietly observing the proximity to death.

## You're My Obsession: Scorpio Season in Focus

We meet Scorpio season in midfall in the Northern Hemisphere, as leaves continue to turn, but more crucially, fall from trees to the ground, crunching under our feet, filling the air with a slightly sweet rotting scent. Scorpio is a water sign, and the leaves returning to wet soil are the start of a regenerative process that shows us that loss is a chance for new growth; the mulch of transformation is Scorpion terrain.

Now the Sun sets a bit earlier each day. Some of us may cling to the daylight, perhaps rising a bit earlier to relish what we know we're about to lose. Nature is showing us that change is not just possible but necessary for survival. This is a kind of death, a letting go of the seeds, ideas, and initiatory pangs we may have felt in relationships that started in the spring or summer. Sweaters we slipped off late last April are removed from the recesses of our closet to warm us in the chill to come. When it comes to our sexual needs, we may ask ourselves: What do we want to retain and what are we ready to release?

Scorpio season signals that in order to know ourselves, our bodies, and our desires, we must let go of old identities—and let them die. It may seem strange to discuss death in a book about sex, but there is a lot of potency here. As we lose access to the Sun and embrace the energy of nighttime, we can explore the unseen, the taboo, and the layers that are usually invisible to us.

The previous fixed sign, Leo, anchored us in the middle of endless summer days, and now we enter the time of longer not-quite-winter nights. Darkness begins to beckon as we contemplate the depths of our psyches, perhaps finally willing to explore the deeper caverns of our desire. We can discover who we are sexually when we contemplate the selves and skins we might shed now, like a snake.

In Scorpio season, we can face our deepest and oldest shames and allow them to fall away like dead leaves. We can experiment with desires we may have once judged. We can look squarely at our fears and experiment with taboos. We can meet, face, and embrace what we really, truly, and deeply want. Scorpio season offers us a raw, unbridled intimacy with the self that may be harder to access during the rest of the year.

Born during the season when daylight vanishes early in the Northern Hemisphere, many Scorpios are nightbirds, doing their best creative work as the rest of the world sleeps. Some of them are night owls that love to sleep late in pitch dark rooms with blackout curtains and dark sleeping masks.

Scorpios can be naturally adept at witchcraft; they tend to understand how to conduct alchemical transformations without anyone teaching them how to do this. They may also know intrinsically how to transmute energy into new forms through ritual enactments, the kind that happen when the spirits are out. Scorpios are often associated with vampiric energy and blood pacts. It's no wonder that Halloween, humanity's celebration of thin veils between the material and spiritual worlds, takes place during this potent, powerful astrological season.

In the months after 9/11 in New York City when the city was in utter crisis, it seemed that many of us were going out and getting laid. We began to call it "fucking against dying"—and this is apt Scorpio terminology. This is a kind of transformation—turning one thing into another, terror into ecstasy. With Scorpio energy, we are often on some kind of heightened threshold that can instantly become something else in a way that feels almost like sorcery.

## Get to Know Mars (Again) and Pluto, the Traditional and Modern Rulers of Scorpio

Scorpio is the first sign we've met with both a traditional and modern rulership, helping us to see better into the powerful multiple facets of the sign. Mars, a fiery warrior god, gives Scorpio its inherent passion and seeming ferocity. As we've discussed, Mars energy is often forward-thrusting. Although Scorpios pursue what they want quite differently than Aries, the other sign ruled by Mars, they do push just as hard as their Mars-ruled sibling sign—it's simply that this force is internalized. The Aries Mars will animalistically assert its desire, but once sex is acquired or denied, they may let it go or grow bored. Scorpio also has a hunting instinct, but their patience is unmatched—they can wait for days, weeks, months, or years for their prey to be perfectly positioned, because Scorpio refuses to miss their mark.

Pluto, the modern ruler of Scorpio, provides a compulsive counterpart, marking Scorpio desire with an obsessive, spiritually transformative quality. Pluto shows us the subterranean, subconscious forces that drive desire and fear, revealing how we often fear what we desire. Its place in our horoscope can show us where we meet our deepest selves, the layers of our ancestors embedded in our DNA. Because Pluto is a slow-moving, generational planet, its house placement and aspects to other planets weave its narrative of descent through our charts—the sign it's in will not tell us much about our individual lives. But where Mars shows us the internalized power of all things Scorpio, Pluto shows us Scorpio's depth-defying regenerative power. Pluto transits to our personal planets often make us feel like a part of us is dying, and the harder we try to cling to it, the more intense its disintegration will be.

## Scorpio's Erotic Gifts

Scorpio, like other signs, is burdened with some pop-astrology stereotypes, and I want to take a moment to say that Scorpios are not "sluts," nor are they "sex fiends" or particularly promiscuous. Any individual Scorpio could exhibit some of these traits with no shame but, if anything, Scorpios might be *less* promiscuous than other signs because they take their desires so seriously.

Part of Scorpio's essential erotic gift is drawn from their powerful attunement to the depths of the human psyche. For them, sexual experiences, whether they're within the bonds of a long-term monogamous relationship, a one-night stand, ethically non-monogamous relationship(s), or a solo sex session, can feel utterly consuming and life-giving. This isn't just sensual pleasure for pleasure's sake, like Taureans, their opposite sign, often experience, but likely an entire in-and-out-of-body experience. The meeting of the genitals can mean a meeting of the mind and soul for Scorpios. Another rare trait possessed by Scorpios is the ability to draw on a psychic bank of power supplied from past sexual experiences over and over again, even years later. The memory lodged in the psyche can be enough for a Scorpio to fully relive an experience in a way that feels very real, providing not just fodder for masturbatory fantasy but making it feel like they're with that person again in real life. These regenerative skills can come in handy when a Scorpio finds themselves without a partner, or if a lover is going through an intentionally celibate phase.

Similarly, Scorpios can experience heightened states of arousal and pleasure from the seemingly smallest erotic exchanges, for instance, kissing. The ability to focus like a laser beam on a singular element, for instance, a lover's mouth, can make it feel like nothing else exists but this erotic exchange, right here, right now. This kind of obsessive, microscopic homing in on a singular sensation is also possible during solo sex. Scorpio's fixation with living each moment as if it's their last can lend heightened intensity to all erotic experiences. This is part of what makes them so memorable.

There can be a sorcerer-like sexual quality to Scorpio people, in the sense that journeying to the underworld (and back, hopefully) is a task they might take to more easily than others. Some astrologers liken Scorpio to Charon, the mythological Greek ferryman who carried the dead across the river Styx. Many Scorpios relish their role as an erotic shaman, and even if they're not playing with BDSM energy, they might thoroughly enjoy taking charge of a lover's psychospiritual sexual experience. Yes, we've debunked the myth about Scorpios as some kind of sex fiend, but an appreciable number of them don't actually mind the rumor.

Subterranean spaces and so-called subversive experiences can be easier for Scorpios to navigate, even if they identify on the vanilla end of the sexual spectrum. Certain Scorpios might feel comfortable at a sex party observing, but not necessarily participating. Scorpios, going against the grain of their pop astrology reputation, can be less experimental than other signs. This sometimes has to do with their emotional vulnerability, as it may be too overwhelming to take on the energy of lots of other people. A Scorpio may focus instead on one or two intense sexual connections across their lifetime. This is not to say that some Scorpios won't indulge in one-night stands or casual sexual dalliances, however.

Many Scorpios would rather fall hard, all the way, into an obsessive, singular love where sex connects and cements their psychospiritual bond. Once a Scorpio is bonded in a monogamous pairing, they can be more likely to remain faithful and not want to change the terms of the relationship at a later date. Outside of ethically non-monogamous relationships, a Scorpio who ventures beyond their primary pair bond sometimes does so because they've been hurt so badly they feel as if the relationship is no longer reparable.

## Pathway to Play and Creativity for Scorpio

Art that transmutes and transgresses is Scorpio art, and if it changes the viewer and the artist at the same time, even more so. Playing with anything that changes a Scorpio as they create it, but that also has the potential to change the *consumer* of the artwork—that's the Scorp sweet spot. Anything from painting to dance to poetry to improv can stir their creative cauldron, but one simple way to transmute matter daily is through kitchen witchery. Cooking for oneself or for a lover is a powerful way to tap into the Scorpion drive to transform. Chopping, simmering, spicing, and metamorphosing the matter of vegetables into a delicious soup to serve may not seem like an obvious erotic endeavor, but gastronomy can definitely be arousing for them.

## Scorpio's Erotic Challenges

*Intense.* That word is all too often associated with Scorpios to the point of cliché—but it's apt, especially in cases where this sign senses their power is threatened. This is why a Scorpion stings, after all—usually because they feel exposed, not because they're actively hunting for prey. When it comes to sex and sexuality, that intensity can go up about a thousand notches. When intimacy is freely given but then imperiled, a Scorpio can feel as if they're losing control.

Scorpio's overwhelming emotional responses can make having and maintaining healthy shared sexual experiences challenging. Paranoia, jealousy, and fear that partners may leave them might cause a Scorpio to leave first or shut down emotionally. They might even do this when partners are willing to discuss challenges in a practical way. When emotionally inflamed, logic is not necessarily a Scorpion strong suit.

It can be quite difficult for Scorpios to return to the intimacy of a sexual bond after their trust has been broken. There are deep fears to face—what for some might just be a breakup can feel like a death to a Scorpio.

What stymies them erotically is the expectation of a trust breach that may come in the future. In some ways, this fear can hover over all their intimate relationships. Then, when an insignificant crack shows up in an intimate relationship, they may simply flee, because in their hearts they always knew this would happen.

What does fleeing intimacy look like for a Scorpio? It might be deleting all traces of an ex's social media, their texts, emails, and phone numbers, burning their love letters, and perhaps something that smacks of revenge. If that happens, it's probably just an instinctual self-protective measure for the Scorpio.

Hiding out for self-protection is something Scorpios are adept at. They can sequester themselves in the shadows and cut themselves off from potentially fulfilling erotic connections with others, just to avoid being hurt or exposing parts of themselves that they've labeled "bad." Libras can make their secret selves invisible by flooding a crowded room with their beauty and charm, but Scorpios seem to hide out in shadowy corners, where they can grow lonely—their fixed water turning to ice. There's nothing wrong with taking time off from romantic or sexual relationships and experimenting with celibacy to figure out what your desires are, but Scorpio must do this consciously and purposefully—not as a form of self-flagellation.

Working through the challenges of being in a complicated relationship or exploring sexuality that feels less than safe means getting hurt is always possible. Unlike their Mars sibling Aries, who tends to burn quickly through their anger, Scorpios can hold grudges that end up hurting them more than those they loved and lost (or pushed away).

Delayed ejaculation, vaginismus, and anorgasmia can result from a Scorpion emotional shutdown. In order to cope with their erotic challenges, Scorpio must find an inner ease to soften their radical, relentless introspection—and stop blaming their emotional distress on others, including lovers, family, and friends. How can they do this? By confronting their fears more gently and lovingly, peeling back their layers more softly, and remembering that even if someone they love leaves, they will never be alone.

## Scorpio Shame and Shadow Work

Because of Scorpio's deep well of emotional sensitivity and rulership over the genitals, they can suffer greatly when raised in households where sex is considered a sin. We must acknowledge that as a baseline, the culture of the United States as simultaneously sex negative and sex obsessed is confusing and often harmful, even to those of us from incredibly progressive backgrounds. But this shame and toxicity is amplified when a Scorpio grows up in a home where their guardian(s) fail to teach them that their body is safe to explore. There can be a loud feedback loop to the genitals, a message that these body parts, specifically because they are able to bring us pleasure, are dangerous to us and others. That feedback loop can grow more and more distorted over time, especially if a Scorpio receives the message that self-touch is an "ungodly" activity. Because of this, they may have even more healing and unpacking to do than other signs. In this way, it can take a lot of time and work to become truly comfortable with their sexual selves, even as they hide their fears and show a tough exterior, flexing their stingers.

Scorpios attune to the genital region of the body and a lot of their energy is directed there. If they were told their desires were shameful or bad early in their life, they may have to do some deep work before they can engage in what feels good to them without guilt. When energy and awareness naturally flow toward the genitals even during nonsexual situations, as it tends to do for Scorpios, shame often follows. Understanding that vaginas, vulvas, anuses, and penises are no different in their intrinsic value than livers, elbows, or toes is important for them—except insofar as consent is required for touch. A Scorpio who develops a healthy relationship with masturbation at a young age will know how to manage their drive and regularly release this energy so that it's not obsessively projected onto their partners or other fetish items.

One of my clients, Beth, a cis woman in her late fifties, was raised in a Mormon household with five siblings. She was the only one who left Utah for college. When she booked a session with me, she had just come out as a lesbian and was newly dating via app in New York City. She had been married to a man from her hometown since the year after graduation—they met as freshmen. The entire time she'd been married, before and after having her three now-grown children, she could only have orgasms when she fantasized about women, but immediately afterward she would often cry. Yet she dutifully stayed in her marriage, never even considering leaving until she became an empty nester and started having perimenopausal panic attacks.

Beth had "left" home and her religion's values—those of modesty, heterosexuality, monogamy, and the subordination of women—she raised her kids in the suburbs near Manhattan and considered herself progressive, teaching her kids to be respectful of other cultures, genders, and sexualities. She even called herself a "recovering Mormon." Yet she packed away her own desires so completely that no one who knew her had any idea that she was attracted to women. Even though she encountered her fears and desires about her sexuality every day and night, she hid them well. When she told her husband, whom she loved as a person, that she was leaving, he was shocked, as were her children and friends. But she had woken up one morning and felt as if she would die if she kept on living this lie and never had the experience of being with a woman. Her obsession with what she wanted was present for years, but it was completely locked down. Her circumstances were such that ENM was not an option, and her values were such that cheating was anathema—so the only thing to do was leave.

Through sex coaching, she sought validation about her sexuality and her choices, but also instruction on dating protocols and the mechanics of sex. She told me that when she was a child of maybe ten or eleven, her mother found her masturbating under her covers. She screamed at her, told her she was going to hell, and punished her severely. She learned not just that her genitals were a source of shame, fear, and potential violence but that the fantasy she was having about another girl at school was to blame for the harsh punishment she received. The broader culture she was raised in was full of these messages too, but being rebuked and punished so directly in a moment of intimacy with her body set in motion decades of lying to herself.

Taurus, Scorpio's opposite sign and shadow, can help Scorps to encounter their inverted self, which can be equally terrifying and revelatory. Taurus energy can muscle its way through complicated emotional situations and sensually indulge in pleasure without fear. How does a vulnerable Scorpio learn from this so they can experience sensual, spiritual sex tethered by the emotional security they crave? By letting go without force, which might look like gently exhaling and letting their bodies feel into the protection of self-generated softness. By knowing they will be okay if their lover ever leaves them or is taken away from them by circumstance. By coming back to what they knew when they were born into a Scorpio body—that everything transmutes eventually, and this is just a healthy part of the cycle of life.

## Journal Questions for Scorpio Shadow Work

- What would happen if I lit up the darkness within me?
- What would happen if I allowed someone I once cut off back in?
- What am I guarding against?
- What if I let that guard down?
- Who do I trust and why?
- What is my deepest, most secret desire?

## A Deeper Look at Body Rulership and Erogenous Zones for Scorpio

Scorpio governs all channels of elimination in the body—what we must let go of to allow our cells to renew themselves. When it comes to the bladder, the bowels, the skin, and other pathways of elimination, before our body expels toxins or whatever else is not needed, it must transform those substances into another kind of matter. This is the principal purpose of Scorpio-ruled systems. Yet we must remember that all these processes can involve shame and secrets. In many cultures our genitals are thought of as "dirty." Our bathrooms, where we urinate and defecate, are places we keep our activities mostly secret, even from lovers.

Scorpio-ruled genitals are governed by the root chakra—the chakra connected to security and safety. This chakra is located at the base of the spine at the perineum, between the genitals and the anus (see diagram on page 19). It's connected with feeling grounded and safe in the world. (Note that some astrologers believe Scorpio can also be associated with the sacral chakra that governs pleasure, and there can of course be overlap in these designations.) Fight-or-flight responses are thought to be held in the root chakra, and this tells us in part why safety and security are so important to Scorpios in relationships (and otherwise).

Practicing self-touch that feels safe and secure first is a wonderful way for Scorpios to build a healthy, loving relationship with their desire principle and create a fulfilling orgasmic response. Before masturbating, repeating the affirmation "I am safe" may seem simple, but it can be an extremely powerful practice.

## An Embodiment Exercise for Scorpio Season

### Exploring Descent and Desire

Sit or lie down, ideally in a room where you have some kind of sacred space, such as an altar or a yoga mat—it should be somewhere you can tune into your interior self. Close your eyes if comfortable and take three to five long, deep, slow breaths from your sacrum to your crown. As you inhale, imagine you are breathing in love. As you exhale, envision that you are releasing pain, stress, and exhaustion.

Imagine yourself at the edge of a beautiful body of water. This might be an ocean, a river, a lake, or a pool. You are alone and naked and feel no shame. Look at the water first, imagine what's below, but then bravely close your eyes. Dive into the water.

Let your body unfurl as the water takes you. Give up any resistance, any need to tread, to open your eyes and see what's there. Just let go and at first, float. Eventually you will begin sinking. Imagine that the water is a kind of holy Scorpio water with magical properties. Let go of any tension in your body. Feel the sensation of floating even though you're deep in the depths, as if you are weighted by an anchor that's taking you perhaps to the very bottom, but that whenever you want, whenever it gets to be too much, you can release it and rise back up to take a breath. As you slowly, ever so slowly descend, begin listening to your heart.

Begin feeling the sensation of the water on your skin. Tune into the way your entire body feels. What organ, limb, or muscles feel awake; what is numb or asleep? What are you feeling in your genitals?

Now tune into your desire, to your relationship with your own body, to your sexuality (not to a partner's sexuality—only to yourself for now). Just listen as you continue to descend. Feel any sensation and note whether any wisdom emerges from the depths.

Continue to descend unless you feel any discomfort or fear. If that happens, remember that you can immediately return to shore. You don't even have to retrace your path: you can instantly rocket yourself to dry land at any moment and end the ritual.

If you can keep going down and down, do so. Descend as deep as you can, letting yourself be infinitely vulnerable in the arms of the water. Whenever you're ready, choose to slowly rise through the water until you sense the light at the surface. Emerge and return to shore. Take up to five additional deep breaths: open your eyes. You are safe.

Ask yourself: What part of my sexual self is dying, or what part must die in order for me to find out what I desire?

## Try These Tools to Connect with Scorpio Energy:

- Try gentle impact play with a partner using a low-impact flogger.

- Take a hand mirror and observe your genitals up close, then write about them, using positive affirmations to describe them.

- Learn how to squirt.

- Talk to a death doula or read books about death, grief, and loss.

- Embrace all your kinks and discover more of them.

# 10

## Sagittarius Sexuality

### Exploration and Enlightenment

these hips
are free hips.

**Lucille Clifton**
"homage to my hips"

**Dates:** November 21–December 21

**Sexual Archetype:** The Eternal Student

**Motivation:** Experience

**Symbol:** The Archer

**Planetary Ruler:** Jupiter (also rules Pisces)

**Element:** Fire

**Modality:** Mutable

**Erogenous Zones and Body Rulership:** The Butt,
Hips, Thighs, and Sciatic Nerve

Healthy Sagittarius energy is bright, big and bold, free, wild and wise, ecstatic, excessive, hilarious, opinionated, adorably awkward, open-minded, and inspirational. As a corrective to the intense dead-seriousness of Scorpio energy, Archers sometimes seem like they were born to laugh uproariously while the world burns, spreading joy like wildfire.

When at their best, the main Sagittarius mission is to have a hell of a good time and to learn something while doing it. Their erotic gift is their generosity, but until they learn to receive as well as they give, they can tumble into tumultuous sexual territory.

Sagittarius craves divine ecstasy and seeks wild abandon. Its main calling is to be *free*. In the sexual realm, this can mean the freedom to fully inhabit their bodies, explore their lovers' bodies, and probe every possibility. When they try to nail down a singular turn-on, they often learn that they're into *everything*. But seeking out every erotic potential can sometimes leave them unfulfilled, because they move on to greener pastures before they experience the entire erotic harvest at hand.

Archers seem to have boundless, explosive vitality, even when they're older and have "slowed down." Sagittarians of all genders tend to express a healthy level of uncontainable confidence. With all three fire signs, Aries, Leo, and Sag, erotic energy can be so active that you can practically see it crackling in the air. But by the time we get to Sagittarius, it can feel like it's almost too big to contain. That's Jupiter energy, baby! (More on that in a bit.)

Sagittarians have *opinions*, and they often get off on providing enlightenment. This is part of their generous nature. They might seem to visually expand into the space around them as they share wisdom, not realizing how much space they're taking up. They can become transfixed while in this state, as if they're channeling this wisdom from elsewhere in the solar system, or at least from an ancient culture whose texts they had the opportunity to mine.

Yet only one sign merges its lower animal half with a human upper body, bringing the rational, philosophical, and thoughtful into kinship with its untamed spirit: Sagittarius, the freedom seeker. With its half-horse, half-human symbol, Sagittarians are more singularly connected to their bodies than most other signs, and this horse-human cannot help but break into an inspirational trot, always seeking the wider expanses.

## Are You Experienced? Sagittarius Season in Focus

As Sagittarius season begins in the Northern Hemisphere, the nippiness outside is getting real. Peak fall foliage is over and trees wave their bare branches at the cold sky, as if to call out, "How long must I wait until spring?" The fire signs/seasons end with Sagittarius. It's important to pause here and consider what this means for Sagittarius as a sign and a season. If we think of Aries as a match at the moment of striking and Leo as the sustained and contained warmth of a bonfire that draws everyone's gaze, we might imagine Sagittarius as a wildfire (emphasis on the WILD) blowing in every direction at once, blazing through unfamiliar territory without fear or favor.

When we get to the last element in any series, the word "evolved" is a useful framework, as the element (fire, in this case) matures as it travels through the seasons. In Sagittarius season we can ask ourselves: What is fire, in the sexual sense, in its last evolutionary stage?

Sagittarius is a finisher in another way—as the third and final of the autumnal signs, it is the bridge to the quieter, icier early winter ahead. This may be why they're one of the funniest signs of all: they're prepping us for the time when we really need to get serious to survive the cold. Their zodiac neighbor, Capricorn, is better known for a dry wit, but Sagittarius can do loud cackling and roll on the floor, exhausting laughter that requires every muscle in the body.

In Sagittarius season, sweaters are on, fireplaces are lit, and holiday lights and tree stands are beginning to pop up on street corners (at least in New York City, where I live). It feels festive. Christmas may not be until Capricorn season, but Sagittarius season is Christmas PARTY season.

Our bodies are beginning to sense that an enforced slowdown and hibernation phase is soon to come, and many of us respond by moving toward excess. This is the season of overdoing it and not worrying about regretting it the next day (for example, potentially hooking up with your colleague at the office Christmas party after too much eggnog). The days are shorter, reminding us that life, too, is short, and we should live a little.

## Get to Know Jupiter, the Planetary Ruler of Sagittarius

Jolly Jupiter, the Greater Benefic and the biggest, boldest planet, is fifth from the Sun. This gas giant is named for the glorious Roman counterpart to the Grecian Zeus, King of the Gods. He's got BPE (Big Planet Energy), and he shows up swinging his prowess around, letting us know there's enough for everyone. Jupiter's offering is abundance. It's considered the planet of luck, bounty, and expansion, giving Sagittarians their noblesse oblige and endless optimism. "Bigger is always better" is Jupiter's mantra.

As much as having auspicious Jupiter around feels good, and may help us win the Powerball (or at least think we can), this planet's other adage is "too much is never enough," and it often just doesn't know when to stop. *Never Too Much* by Luther Vandross is one of this planet's many theme songs (he can't choose just one; he needs a whole playlist). Jupiter, by transit or natal placement, can show us that you actually *can* have too much luck. When does pleasurable indulgence become a dangerous addiction? That's something Jupiter can't answer, because his mouth is full and he's too busy inhaling the entire buffet of life in one sitting. (When we meet Saturn in the next chapter, he'll give us a plan for that.)

## Sagittarius' Erotic Gifts

Optimism and joy are usually stupendous assets in the bedroom, and Sagittarius comes with generous portions of both. Exuberance creates a genuine curiosity about new experiences that can fuel the Sagittarian sexual spirit. Being naturally inquisitive, candid, and unafraid to ask embarrassing questions can lead to immensely satisfying sexual encounters, especially as they have the ability to laugh at awkward situations, sexual and otherwise. They have a way of self-soothing with humor, making the phrase "laughter is the best medicine" a tool they can employ in their lives every day.

When their sexuality is allowed to flourish, Sagittarians can be the quintessential "Trysexuals" of the zodiac, in the "I'll try anything once" sense. This experimental, curious approach to sex often allows Sagittarians to take life and love less seriously, leading to unanticipated erotic encounters. Archers come in bold, but they often sense that there is no such thing as "too big to fail," and they may intentionally get into awkward situations just in case they might turn out great. An outsized confidence belies their tendency to trip and fall into bed—sometimes literally (because they slipped on their lover's panties or something). The Sagittarius fire is not about showing off, as it may be with Leo, or rushing to the finish line, as it might be for Aries—it's just curiosity about what might happen next, with few designs on the outcome.

This confidence can present as a healthy body image and a willingness to get naked often. Sagittarians who've done their shadow work tend to crave experience above all else, and love to try things so that they have stories to tell. Maybe like that time they accidentally ended up at a sex party after they met that guy at the bar and he introduced them to his friend and then they tried a strap-on for the first time and discovered that they loved it. Sagittarian stories are fantastic and often take unexpected turns!

Thanks to impulsive, expansive, big-mouthed Jupiter, Sagittarians often say exactly what's on their mind without reservation, even in sexual situations. This can be a bit shocking at first to new lovers, and even throw established partners for a loop, but knowing that it's all on the table without subterfuge can provide more pleasure for all involved. That is the glorious erotic feedback loop of Sagittarius.

## Pathway to Play and Creativity for Sagittarius

Creative endeavors that deepen and expand worldly knowledge are the most inspirational and alive for Sagittarians. Becoming a storyteller by reading voraciously is one of the most enlightening projects an Archer can take on. Even if they can't see the world, at least they can read about it and go on journeys on the page. A deep, consistent daily journaling practice is also undeniably meaningful—note that journey and journaling have the same root. Taking this deeper by journaling about desire, erotic longings, and sex—that's an ideal pathway to Sagittarian play.

## Sagittarius' Erotic Challenges

Even lucky Jupiter-ruled Sagittarians can experience discomfort and trauma—all survivors of nervous-system dysregulating stress need grounded, practical coping strategies. The Sagittarian response to feeling weird or uncomfortable might be to barrel through or try to find philosophical answers, or move on quickly to something else, perhaps a lover who seems to have all the answers. Sometimes they'll choose partners with big egos and little substance and perform the role of an acolyte for these folks. They may fall for a grifter-guru because they project their quest for knowledge onto them, as if they've found some kind of holy sex god. What Sagittarius needs to do is find the sex god within.

It may be challenging to fully develop their own erotic map and carve out a clear path for their desire, because they often crave constant change. It's tricky to navigate whether boredom with a particular partner is legitimately hurting their libido, or if they're running away to avoid the deeper wisdom of their heart and body. Sexually, Sagittarius can be open and experimental, but sometimes they are almost *too* curious, in the sense that boredom can be an ever-present possibility.

Commitment to a relationship can be challenging for Sagittarius, unless they cement their independence first and feel free within its constraints. If a sexual partner expects too much or demands anything that feels contractual or smacks of domestic obligation, Archers may withdraw and shut down or continue to search for lover(s) who understand and respect their quest for freedom. This, ideally, is a conversation a Sagittarius should be willing to have at the outset of a relationship.

The Sagittarius search for Eternal Truth can end up stymying their sexual growth and expansion. They can get so fervently caught up in chasing enlightenment that they forget that their own commonplace desires are worth exploring, too.

## Sagittarius Shame and Shadow Work

Where Virgo, the previous mutable sign, sees the individual trees, Sagittarius considers the whole forest and its growth. Yet when a Sag encounters cultural or familial decrees about religion, ethics, or morals that they can't break free from, sometimes the search for meaning never takes off in the first place. The polarity between Sagittarius and their opposite sign is stark: even though they're both mentally agile, mutable signs, Gemini collects data and Sagittarius translates; the former is concerned with facts, while the latter craves meaning and eschews details.

Shadow work for Sagittarius can require an honest (a favorite Archer word) interrogation of their own dogma. Where have beliefs that once led to paradigm shifts calcified into judgments of others who disagree? Where does early childhood indoctrination, particularly for those raised in a religious home, still have a hold on sexuality and body image right now?

Understanding one's sexuality is complicated enough, but adding a layer of ideology can complicate it even more. Ironically, Sagittarius, one of the most liberated signs, can carry secret yet powerful patriarchal shame into their sexual relationships—even when they're in open, poly, or otherwise non-mainstream partnerships.

And then there is the other side—reacting against patriarchal conditioning and falling so deeply into an "alternative" sexual philosophy that it becomes the one and only truth. For example, the philosophy of tantra, a Hindu and Buddhist tradition developed in India, can, as a study and practice, be an enlightening, rich, and pleasurable pursuit. But a Sagittarius avoiding their shadow work can become so obsessed and enmeshed with tantric teachings that they can blot out everything else, including the feelings they used to have for a particular lover. They might entirely leave their life behind and join a sex cult (or just a regular cult) if they think they have found the singular answer to everything. A few months or years later, once that projection breaks, it can be devastating for the Sag who believed with their whole soul that they had found the One True Answer. When challenged, Sagittarians can default to a sense of self-righteousness. Gemini asks Sagittarius, "How do you really know what you think you know? Have you actually looked at the data?"

Amy, a queer cis woman and Sagittarius Sun in her late thirties, had made the pursuit of different kinds of lovers into almost a second career in her twenties. She lived out her dream of sex with an extraordinary number of humans from every walk of life, gender, and proclivity. Although she was a deeply curious, intelligent person, she had dropped out of college and abandoned plans to study theology abroad.

On the three occasions she fell in love in her thirties, with the idea of "settling down," it was with abusive partners that convinced her they had all the answers. Each one of them had a guru complex, and she believed she would learn the secrets to life as their partner. These men acted all-knowing and spoke in sermons, as if their declarative sentences, no matter how messy and frankly wrong they were, were the final answer to all questions that might ever be asked.

Although she had made a habit of relentlessly and guiltlessly pursuing sexual pleasure before, these men refused to provide it for her, and it wasn't until after leaving the last of these relationships that she realized she hadn't orgasmed the entire time she was with him. After she escaped her first relationship with an abuser who hid his violence in a cloak of Buddhism, she fell for a musician who had a fanatical female following but secretly believed women shouldn't have jobs. He ghosted her when she talked about going back to school to finish her degree. Finally, she met and was devastated by a man who fancied himself the business version of Tony Robbins. He spoke in aphorisms, never introduced her to his family, and essentially indoctrinated her into his cult. He forbade her from masturbating for several months of their relationship—claiming that it would be a healthy form of "fasting."

She broke free after two years with the help of friends who staged an intervention. That's how she ended up in a session with me. We quickly identified the problem—she had subjugated her own curiosity and desire for adventure and projected it onto each of these partners in unique ways. She not only gave up her autonomy and desire for sexual exploration, she entirely neglected her own emotional needs in service to their demands, forgetting who she was and what she wanted. During session one, she realized that not only did she not experience orgasms with these partners—she barely laughed.

We worked together over six months to restore her confidence, help her find her joy, and remind her that the answers she was looking for were within her all along. She began dating and having sexual adventures again, and she connected with a loving partner who respected her mind and cared deeply for her heart, body, and soul; their open relationship, at this time, is still going strong.

Getting to the heart of Sagittarian shadow work can be tricky because Archers may think they've found the one and only true answer many times over during their journey into the depths of their sexual selves. Making sure their big questions are answered with enough honesty and clarity and a uniquely personal response instead of a philosophical treatise is part of the work. Letting the mind become quiet and still, and slowing down enough to take in the many truths of their existence is a challenge, especially if that feels like settling for one idea of what love and sex should mean. When they allow pure joy to fuel this journey, they can get there faster and stay there longer.

## Journal Questions for Sagittarius Shadow Work

- What am I running away from?
- What facts about my erotic self would I like to avoid?
- What would happen if I stood still?
- Why am I running away, and what am I running toward?
- Is anyone enough for me?
- Am I enough for myself?

## A Deeper Look at Body Rulership and Erogenous Zones for Sagittarius

Sagittarius rules the hips, thighs, and butt. The muscles of the thighs are what propel many of us forward—they enable walking and running, and also running away from things (and people) that Sagittarians believe are holding them back from exploring. Keeping these muscles healthy, supple, and strong, as much as you are able, is a wise Sagittarian strategy. Consider honoring these body parts during Sagittarius season, or all year long if you have placements in Sagittarius. A simple way to draw attention to this part of the body is to practice rolling your hips and doing hip circles throughout the day. Another fun way to honor Sagittarius energy is to accentuate your own hips and butt in the way you dress, even showing a bit of strategic thigh in appropriate moments. Curves and Sagittarius go well together.

During solo sex, focus on hip thrusting, varying between slow and fast movements. The late, great sex educator Betty Dodson, iconic author of *Sex for One* and a masturbation mentor to millions, taught vulva-owners how to raise their hips while self-pleasuring, and it's a spot-on Sagittarian strategy. In partnered sex, you might focus on foreplay that involves stroking, kissing, and caressing a lover's hips, thighs, and butt, and encourage partners to pay attention to these areas of your body. Gently grabbing and squeezing a partner's hips during sex can also be satisfying—this can also be a fun invitation to sex, or just cuddling.

Sagittarians are often wildly turned on when a lover pays attention to the insides of their thighs, especially with small kisses that start at the knees and work their way up toward the genital area, and they may want to practice this on their lovers as well. Experimenting with cowboy and reverse cowboy, or any position that evokes the sensation of being ridden or riding a lover, or alternating between being the horse and the rider, can be super fun and wildly erotic. Consider making the butt a main feature of sexual encounters—as in making it a high-visibility area and showing it off by having sex from behind. For more intimacy, you can stimulate Sagittarian erogenous zones by sitting up, with your thighs on top of a lover's, and calves wrapped around their back, with your hands on one another's hips.

## An Embodiment Exercise
## for Sagittarius Season

### Laughing Meditation to Awaken Desire

This meditation takes about ten minutes. If available to you, stand and place your feet hip-width apart, stretching your arms over your head. Rock your hips from side to side, then do a few small hip circles, gently moving in a way that feels good. If you can comfortably touch your toes, do so, or just stretch toward them, then slowly and gently rise back up, stretching your arms over your head again. Yawn, massage, and move your jaw, slowly and gently. You may sit or stand to perform the meditation, whatever feels best!

Close your eyes, and begin by smiling a bit, then laugh quietly for a minute or two. At first, you might just be making the sounds and vibrations of laughter, which may feel forced, but as you continue, it can begin to feel much more natural.

Now get louder until you're creating deep, powerful belly laughs—it's okay if these feel forced at first. Put your hands on your belly to see how this feels and continue for a few minutes laughing from your deepest core. Keep laughing, moving back to smaller, quieter laughter, then moving back to the deep belly laughter again, as if you're making laughter circles.

Notice which parts of your body are activated. Are you feeling joy or desire anywhere? Move your hands to any part of the body that feels awakened, enlivened—likely the belly—but this could be any part of you. Now move your arms to sweep that activated energy toward your hips and thighs, or toward your genital region. You might also visualize this energy as orange light traveling from one region of the body to another.

If it feels right, using a toy or your hand, pleasure yourself, noticing whether after the laughter this feels different from "average" solo sex sessions.

## Try These Tools to Connect with
## Sagittarius Energy:

- Experiment with outdoor sex (keep it legal and safe, please).

- Book a hotel room alone to enliven your solo sex life, even just for a night, or ask if you can stay at a friend's place when they're away from home.

- Learn belly dance or twerking (ideally from the people who created these art forms).

- Read *Urban Tantra: Sacred Sex for the Twenty-First Century* by Barbara Carrellas.

- Discover new comedians—the raunchier the better.

# 11

# Capricorn Sexuality

## Discipline and Determination

Nature does nothing without purpose or uselessly.

**Aristotle**

*Politics*

**Dates:** December 21–January 21

**Sexual Archetype:** The Authority

**Motivation:** To Be Useful

**Symbol:** The Sea Goat

**Planetary Ruler:** Saturn (also rules Aquarius)

**Element:** Earth

**Modality:** Cardinal

**Erogenous Zones and Body Rulership:** The Skin,
Joints, Bones, Teeth, and Knees

Healthy Capricorn energy is self-disciplined, cautious, wise, mature, formidable, grounded, protective, pragmatic, surprisingly sensual, and ultra-powerful. Caps know how to go the distance and can be complete masters of time—their own and others. Sexually, they're often willing to work harder than other signs, yet their sex lives can suffer when they're too hard on themselves. They may live under the false belief that to experience pleasure, they must first achieve a form of greatness, leaving them isolated. Caps need to cultivate a beginner's mind and remember that they deserve to feel good not as a goal to attain but as a given every single day.

I want to debunk a pop astrology theme that runs through many descriptions of Capricorn, colored by a "pull yourself up by your bootstraps" lens. The idea that Goats are fervent financial and corporate strivers who care more about success, money, and their professional goals than relationships, love, family, and sex—this is capitalist claptrap. "Doing the work" doesn't necessarily mean it's the work of attaining wealth or getting the proverbial corner office. Capricorns are complex and creative beings who should not be reduced to how much they've achieved out there in the world. They have a rich inner life, and though they tend to work very, very hard, it's not always about affluence. Once again for the people in the back: not all Caps are capitalists!

Capricorn is signified by The Devil card in the Tarot, but this is *not* a classic representation of evil as good's opposite. Rather, we can better understand Capricorn's connection to Pan, the Greek nature deity, who is essentially the god of the wild. Pan cavorted with nymphs and had dominion over the fields, pastures, and forests. With his goat legs, horns, and hoofs, Pan is the original sex god. In simple terms, early Christians may have seen those hoofs in depictions of Pan and made Capricorn into the devil. When the Tarot was created in Italy in the 1430s and eventually adapted as a fortune-telling tool in France in the 1780s, we began to see the devil we know.

In addition to the unfortunate capitalist associations, the evil devil is a common trope in the modern Capricorn delineation, further souring Caps on their own history and their myriad potentials. There's no need to get stuck in those stereotypes, though, because even a certain type of Capricorn, one who lives a conventional, socially acceptable life, might find that they can be a CEO by day and a sex deity by night. As hardcore and Saturnine as some Caps can be, this is one essential way to connect to their sensuality and let go of striving, just for a moment. The late David Bowie exuded this kind of Capricorn energy.

## Under Pressure: Capricorn Season in Focus

Here we are, at the last cardinal sign, the last earth sign, and the start of the final season of the year before we start all over again in spring. The zodiacal wheel has brought us to a time when we take stock, gather with our loved ones, and reflect on the past year. Christmas, the first holiday of Capricorn season, is a version of Saturnalia, a pagan celebration of the god and planet that rules Capricorn. It's time to come in from the cold and warm your body by the fire, or under the comforter with your lover. We might seek solace in the pleasures of the flesh even more because it's so cold outside. As winter babies, Capricorns understand what it means to have hours and hours of darkness in which to cuddle and play. We might also find ourselves in a more controlled environment, deeply acquainted with the night, and able to experiment and play with power.

The winter solstice, when Capricorn begins, hearkens back to summer's polarity, with the longest day of the year in the Northern Hemisphere giving way to the longest night six months later. A trade-off that is both an ending and a beginning, sexual renewal feels possible now, and setting intentions for intimacy can help us start the year off right. It's a coincidence of the Gregorian calendar that New Year's Eve and its requisite resolutions come during Capricorn season, but it's a useful coincidence nonetheless, and *useful* is one of Capricorn's favorite words. During Capricorn season, we can find ourselves more often in solitude, even if we are partnered. Here we can tease apart what our erotic needs are—what feeds and sustains us—from the kind of erotic energy that feels like something we can live without.

## Meet Saturn, the Planetary Ruler of Capricorn

Ah, Saturn, the most feared, misunderstood of the planets, and one of my absolute favorites to work with. Saturn is considered one of the malefic planets in astrology (the other malefic is Mars). Saturn is the god who ate his children—famously portrayed in Francisco Goya's *Saturn Devouring His*

*Son*, which hangs in the Museo Nacional del Prado in Madrid, Spain. It is a dark and gory portrait of a crazed god tearing his bloodied child limb from limb with his teeth. Google it. That's not the Saturn that I know, though.

Saturn is known as the Cosmic Taskmaster, or as I have affectionately called him, Big Daddy Saturn. His energy can feel harsh, demanding, and sometimes cruel, but this is the kind of planet that has our best interests, growth, and longevity at heart. Daddies, guardians, protectors, saviors—everything (unnecessarily) associated with the concept of "the father" is deeply loaded in our culture, steeped in patriarchy, control, and harmful systems. But stripped down to the bare bones (our bones are ruled by Saturn), this structural energy is simply what holds us up—gives our flesh a shape we can recognize. Saturn's purpose is to help us find our integrity and be our true selves. That's why goal setting is so central to Capricorn season.

## Capricorn's Erotic Gifts

What would our sex lives be without some structure? A string of disconnected experiences that don't necessarily create a lot of meaning and fulfillment. Capricorn is a sign where fantasies can become tangible and actionable. Capricorn's erotic gift is taking sexual impulses, desires, and curiosities and giving them a recognizable shape. When a Cap knows how to own their "nos," everything feels possible.

The waiting is *not* the hardest part for Capricorn—in fact, they tend to be so adept at waiting that it can become a sexual superpower. As masters of time, it's often possible for a Goat to suss out and cultivate a healthy, robust sex life—solo or shared—one that's mature and well worth the wait. This might mean becoming highly sexually skilled or becoming enviably orgasmic, but perhaps not until one's thirties or forties (see the section on the Saturn Return later in this chapter). It also may mean that remaining sexually active through a ripe old age is more than possible—it's probable. This is a sign for whom deep investigations of erotic energy such as studying tantra might intrigue, as it's a practice that may encourage delayed gratification.

Capricorns might seem visibly connected to their bodies even more than their sibling earth signs Taurus and Virgo, thanks to the anchoring energy of Saturn. Even if they're not up for spontaneous sex romps, some Caps can be intrinsically sensual lovers who take their eroticism very seriously. They can be adept at staying present during sex, something other signs struggle with.

A cardinal earth sign, Capricorns may be very willing to initiate and develop a practical and useful sexual skill set. They can come up with erotic concepts and put them into action, then execute them successfully. Fiery Aries, one of the other cardinal signs, tends to burn out after an initial push. But Caps can keep going after they've birthed a creative or sexual idea: they see through the entire process and won't give up until everyone is sated. As masters of both planning and implementation, sexual pleasure, wellness, and satisfaction can become a whole, satisfying, sustaining meal for Capricorns and their lovers.

## Pathway to Play and Creativity for Capricorn

As much as Sagittarius, the previous sign, is a born comedian given to accidental slapstick, hilarious rhetoric, and standup riffs, we should not sleep on the powerful dry humor of the seemingly withholding Capricorn. Goats are extremely funny, in a way that people who have experienced hard times are funny—it's a strategy for dealing with adversity. They are often self-deprecating, especially with new lovers, speaking directly to their sexual skills, almost as a warning in case something goes wrong. Probing and pursuing the roots of their achingly dry wit in public and private, and perhaps even experimenting with improv, can provide unexpectedly joyous paths to play and creativity for Caps. They may also delight in building with their hands, from Lego sets and massive jigsaw puzzles to architectural models and erector sets. Anything that takes time and planning is an excellent artistic endeavor for a Cap.

## Capricorn's Erotic Challenges

One of the biggest erotic challenges for Capricorns is a tendency to feed on stress like it's oxygen. Capricorns may live by the "failure is not an option" adage, which can push the pursuit of pleasure down to the bottom of their to-do list. Stressful situations can almost turn into a kind of comfort for them, simply because they're so good at handling the very things that may drive others mad. If they receive praise, accolades, and gratitude for coming to everyone's rescue, they may take even more on. Yet their inherent skillfulness and focused rationality can only take them so far, especially when it comes to being holistically present in their bodies and erotically connected to others. You can't always dispense with the heart, even when your goal is not romantic love.

Sharon Olds's gorgeous poem "Sex Without Love"[1] feels so very Capricorn and incredibly instructive regarding Caps' tendency to test themselves, crowding out all other needs. In the last stanza, she compares lovers to runners challenging themselves, alone with the road surface and their body, then alone in the universe. It ends with these lines.

> The single body alone in the universe
> against its own best time.

When Capricorn does their work solely for accolades or for any other purpose than being "the single body alone in the universe against its own best time," they can lose themselves and their access to pleasure. Yet at the same time, constructing too many harsh boundaries can drive them to rigidity, brittleness, and a self-perpetuating cycle of loneliness and isolation.

Of all the signs, Capricorns who are less self-aware seem to be most invested in clinging to old, ancestral concepts of guilt and shame. I've found that even Capricorn clients raised in progressive homes without any blatant negative religious messaging about sex somehow find these tropes in the broader culture and take them on as their own. In this way, Saturn, as the Cosmic Taskmaster, can inadvertently create a wall between a Capricorn and their desires, rather than just helping them create healthy boundary-building skills.

# A Note on the Saturn Return

When we near the ages of twenty-nine and a half, fifty-eight, and ninety, we all experience the "Saturn Return"—the astrological transit that occurs every time Saturn completes his journey around the Sun in our lifetime, returning to where it was when we were born. (I co-wrote a book about this phenomenon called *Surviving Saturn's Return: Overcoming the Most Tumultuous Time of Your Life* during my own Saturn Return.) This can be a period of crisis and renewal, and it's particularly affecting for those with a lot of Saturn in their charts—the harsh challenges that are a defining characteristic of Capricorns, as they're ruled by the Cosmic Taskmaster.

As tough as life can be for Caps, after they complete their first Saturn Return, they often feel like they've scaled a very significant mountain. If approached with self-love and integrity, this can lead to a profound realignment and a far deeper level of authentic self-esteem. If they felt old and prematurely wizened when they were chronologically younger, this can give them a chance to experience something that feels like youth again. And if this revelatory experience was missed in their late twenties or experienced as pure hardship with no upside—the middle-aged version of the transit can create the same psychological conditions, making post-midlife a much freer and more joyful time. Essentially, after each Saturn Return, the burden Caps tend to carry can be considerably lightened, as it creates a crucible of intense emotional growth. This phase can set Caps free from the guilt and sexual shame they've carried, especially if they set an intention to do so at the outset of their Saturn Return.

## Capricorn Shame and Shadow Work

Capricorns tend to *consciously think* they want structure, stability, and control in their love and sex lives. Secretly, they often want to have their fears acknowledged, then to be fed, nourished, and swaddled like a baby. That's because their opposite constellation and shadow energy comes from Cancer, a sensitive, intuitive, maternal water sign.

For Capricorn, sometimes reaching into the murky, dark depths where their fear lives is the way to loosen up the access to their pleasure and joy. Pleasure without reflection can feel like an empty vessel for a Cap. Learning how to be alone without being lonely is an essential area of focus for the Capricorn who wants to experience more love and pleasure. It's counterintuitive, surely, that inviting yet more introspection and isolation can create a healthy sex life, but for this sign, it's true. However, being sure to carefully strategize and schedule solo time around quality engagement with partners, friends, family, and others can prevent a collapse into too much isolation.

Mike, a cis man with his Sun and Saturn in Capricorn, eventually came to identify as pansexual in our work together. He had suffered from depression and anxiety for as long as he could remember. When he booked a session with me at the age of twenty-nine, he was enveloped in what he described as the "most intense depression I've ever experienced." The SSRIs he'd been on since he was a late teen were no longer effective, and he was working with his psychiatrist to tweak them, but when he began losing his erection with his partner as his dosage increased, he felt utterly despondent.

He loved his girlfriend of five years, and they got along very well. His ED began to consume all his thoughts, making it difficult to relate to his partner day-to-day. Even though she was comforting and tried to work on communication with him, he created more and more barriers, pushing her away and eventually shutting her out completely, just as the pandemic began. When I first met him via Zoom, she had just moved out. He found himself completely isolated, a victim of despair and loneliness that he knew he had created for himself. Shame about his body had been a running theme in his life, dating back to puberty, when he first realized that his smaller frame was different than the other boys at his school. He inherited the slender, wiry physique of his father, who was rarely at home and consumed with his work.

When he began to display symptoms of depression and anxiety as a teen, Mike was taken directly to the psychiatrist for a medical evaluation—his parents didn't even consider adjunctive therapy. Although they were not a religious family and there were no overtly sex-negative messages in Mike's home, he sensed the coldness between his parents, and their silence about what was wrong spoke louder to him than any words could. When we began working together, it was all catching up with him, all at once.

I told him that we would aim to turn this crisis into a chrysalis by starting with his body image, a crucial but often overlooked Capricorn issue. Over the course of a year, we explored the origins of his body dysmorphia, gave him tools to reclaim his erotic energy and power, like the practices shared in this book, and made space for him to explore identities. He immersed himself in new communities online and safely explored his sexuality using apps like Feeld from the safety of lockdown, eventually discovering that he was attracted to a much wider variety of humans than he'd consciously allowed himself to consider.

By the time he completed his Saturn Return and turned thirty, he emerged from the pandemic, started dating, and explored satisfying sex with partners who looked and felt different than what had previously been compelling to him. He learned how to control his ED using a variety of techniques, from visualization to practicing with a masturbation sleeve, and on the rare occasions he lost an erection with new partners, he no longer found it devastating. He just said, "This happens once in a while, but we can have fun in other ways." And he definitely did!

The Capricorn relationship to shadow is shaped by their very acute relationship with guilt for pursuing pleasure. The sense that they have to work excruciatingly hard to obtain their goals, and only then can they enjoy life (or sex), must be interrogated. Asking themselves, on a daily basis, when and where they can experience pleasure, even before they work, is an integral part of this process. Separating pleasure from pain, even though these two areas of the brain exist on the same pathway, is a major part of unearthing access to what feels good.

## Journal Questions for Capricorn Shadow Work

- What would happen if the scaffolding of my life was dismantled?
- What holds me up?

- What if no one saves me?

- Do I believe I deserve pleasure if I don't work for it?

- What if I actually let someone save me?

- What do I need from a lover or potential lover that I don't have right now? Can I soften and ask for it, even if they may say no?

## A Deeper Look at Capricorn Body Rulership and Erogenous Zones

Capricorn rules our skin, bones, and fascia—the things that keep our meat-sack bodies from melting into a puddle of organic matter on the floor. In this way, there is no outer part of the body that is not an erogenous zone for Caps.

The knees are especially sensitive, and they should be well supported during any positions that require being on them, from doggie style to oral on the side of the bed. Use pillows, knee pads, whatever tends to this sensitive area. Caressing and kissing the knees as a matter of course during foreplay is a go-to for Caps and their lovers.

Capricorn's rulership of the teeth makes biting an intriguing potential turn on. Note that biting a lover gently is one thing, but going for anything harder than a kitten's nip requires consent.

Our bones are wrapped in the fascia that holds our bodies together, but without enough water that fascia can dry up, causing pain that may feel impossible to treat. Capricorns must keep hydrated. And not just by drinking water: using lube liberally is always okay and should be part of a Capricorn sex regimen, solo and partnered. There is a persistent myth that "needing" lube is some kind of failure, and that's one I'd like to bust permanently. Even if you're a vulva-owner who produces ample vaginal lubrication naturally when turned on, learn what lube you like, and keep it in your nightstand. Anyone, at any time, might require a little bit of lube.

## An Embodiment Exercise for Capricorn Season

### Fall in Love with Your Fear

To gain access to Capricorn's limitless arsenal of meaningful, long-lasting sexual pleasure and prowess, first, fears must be faced. This exercise can help you meet your fear in a safe space and begin to send it packing. If you find this too triggering you can always stop, and this is also something you can do in the safe container you work in with your therapist or another counselor.

Lie in bed, where you dream. Take a few deep cleansing breaths and close your eyes if that feels comfortable. Focus on all your muscle groups, first tensing and then relaxing them, starting with your toes and working all the way up to the top of your body. When you're fully relaxed, allow yourself to focus on your biggest boogeyman—your worst, most irrational fear—whether it is a fear of failing in the sexual sense, or something else.

See it in your mind's eye, whatever this monster, devil, guilt-trip, or shame demon looks like.

What is your fear? Say it out loud if you feel safe. Imagine it in vivid detail. But every thirty seconds, even while immersed in this fear, give yourself a little pinch that says, "I am awake, and I have nothing to fear." You can pinch your inner arm, your knee, or anywhere that feels like it will gently prick you.

Continue to walk through the fear scene like it's a Technicolor dream, then give yourself a little pinch. Let yourself feel all that dread, then give yourself a little pinch. When you are finished imagining the worst, forgive yourself for carrying this fear for so long, perhaps across generations, from distant past lives. You are okay—you don't have to carry that fear anymore. In your mind's eye, watch that fear leaving your body in a heavy cloud, then getting lighter and floating to the ceiling, up and out into the universe. Now it is gone.

Using massage oil or another kind of cream, gently massage the part of your body that you have been pinching. Continue to do this and see if it begins to feel sensual, stimulating, or turns you on. If you want to pleasure yourself, go for it!

## Try These Tools to Connect with Capricorn Energy:

- Experiment with age play, where you or a lover role-play that you're significantly older or younger than you currently are.

- Experiment with student/teacher role-playing.

- Try light bondage.

- Google Esther Perel's "Intimacy Inventory" and take it.

- Do a session with a sex coach to help you focus on your sexual goals.

# 12

# Aquarius Sexuality

## Invention and Individuality

There is nothing new under the sun, but there are new suns.

**Octavia E. Butler**

*Parable of the Trickster*

**Dates:** January 21–February 19

**Sexual Archetype:** The Visionary

**Motivation:** Liberation

**Symbol:** The Water Bearer

**Planetary Ruler:** Saturn (Traditional, also rules
Capricorn) and Uranus (Modern)

**Element:** Air

**Modality:** Fixed

**Erogenous Zones and Body Rulership:** The Veins/
Circulation, Electrical Impulses of the Body, Muscles and
Tendons of the Lower Legs, and Ankles

Heathy Aquarius energy is progressive yet rational, brilliant, electric, eclectic, self-possessed, freedom seeking, analytical, altruistic, and utterly unique. When they've done their shadow work, they are geniuses who imagine the future, tinker with it, and signal the rest of us about what's to come. At their best, they're sexually experimental and advanced, but if they close off their hearts and detach from their bodies, they can have a hard time finding erotic fulfillment and the openness they tend to crave.

Note that Aquarius is *not* a water sign, even though its glyph depicts waves. This is the Water *Bearer*—the one who holds the vessel that contains the liquid. It's twice removed, in fact, from the emotional body, which is one of the reasons this sign has a rather detached reputation. Yet there is the promise of *knowing* that the sea of the collective unconscious, the interconnected whole, perhaps the entire cosmos, is there for them if they allow it in.

One issue for Aquarius, sexually, is to connect to the body so that the mind doesn't run away with all the pleasure, filing it away in a box of neurons that fail to provide a stress-releasing corporeal experience.

Like Fox Mulder from *The X-Files* (famously played by a Leo, David Duchovny, an Aquarian opposite), this sign knows that the truth is out there—but to attune to and heal their sexual selves, they must first tend to inner investigations of their own heart and body. Sometimes the natural intimacies of their everyday experiences and relationships are ignored in favor of the complex architecture of the universe itself. Speaking of sci-fi, there are a number of cultural references that can help us understand the sometimes abstract, over-intellectualized, hyper-objective Aquarian realm. The movie *The Matrix* is a kind of Aquarian utopia/dystopia, a place where there are no moving bodies, only minds in suspended animation. This might sound like a happy, or at least interesting, place to a Water Bearer. Another fun one is the animated series *Futurama*, in which one of their returning gags is a room full of famous dead people with their heads suspended in jars, keeping their brains alive, and cracking jokes at each other's expense. Above all else, Aquarius, as a fixed air sign, tends to believe strongly in their visionary ideas and wants them to reach all of humanity, especially when they have an unconventional edge.

## Get Ur Freak On: Aquarius Season in Focus

We're in the deep freeze now in the Northern Hemisphere. We may slip on icy ground as our hot breath turns to fog, if we dare to step outside, that is. If we're lucky, we're tethered to warm, indoor spaces, and we may slow down our bodies in favor of moving our brains. The middle of winter, the core of the season, can feel like an infinite place for our minds and the ideas they imagine.

Yes, winter can be depressing with its short days and harsh winds. But it calls for grand observations and experiments, making us all into little Nietzsches (Friedrich had Saturn and Neptune in Aquarius) trying to find a solution for our collective pain, or scientists tinkering with ways to survive these dark, cold days. I'm looking at you, Ray Kurzweil (computer scientist and creator of the concept of the singularity) and Michio Kaku (theoretical physicist)—both Aquarius Suns. Because our worlds are effectively made smaller by the cold and ice, we may crave intellectual expansion now. Books provide this, and for the last three decades, we've had the internet.

During Aquarius season, sexual experimentation can help us advance to a "next level" of self-awareness about our desires, even when those desires might make us uncomfortable. In a moment of isolation, when we're separated from our usual peer group and alone in the dark, away from the people we act like, talk like, dress like, and tend to emulate, we may find that our desires are less socially sanctioned, at least in the heteronormative world. Yet we might find peer groups online that allow us to intellectually explore the possibilities.

Certainly not all Aquarians are queer, but queerness as a transgressive concept has always felt very Aquarian to me. Aquarius is about the interconnection of all things, distinctly different but united to form a whole. Aquarius as a community connector finds broken pieces or square pegs and brings them together, so everyone sees that they're facets of a rainbow, and their differences should be celebrated. Aquarius is also where society's outcasts, those who feel like aliens, come together and form community. Aquarius season is a lovely time to find and connect with the people who may one day be your chosen family.

## Get to Know Saturn (Again), the Traditional Planetary Ruler of Aquarius

Most of the details about Saturn can be found in the Capricorn chapter, because these two next-door neighbor signs share this planetary ruler. But in Aquarius, Saturn takes on a different vibe. Where Capricorn's version of Saturn can be earnest and melancholy—in search of something to make THEIR lives meaningful and important, and perhaps their progeny's lives as well—Aquarius seeks to make ALL of life on Earth meaningful. When it rules Aquarius, Saturn takes on the burden of fixing all of society's ills.

The lens widens here, and Saturn starts looking toward the future instead of mainly focusing on the past or building a legacy for their epitaph. Saturn is still our celestial timekeeper in Aquarius, marking our short stay on Earth, but in Aquarius, we can begin to think about Saturnian time differently. In Capricorn, Saturn offers us time that feels linear as we look at our past and work toward a goal: this is a traditional view of time as a marker of history. In Aquarius, time feels far less linear, almost like a neural network of space-time, where Everything Is Happening Everywhere All at Once. (Another movie reference for you here if you haven't seen the brilliant sci-fi film directed by Daniel Kwan.)

Saturn is still cold and strict in Aquarius, but he begins to break through the boundaries that were built to fit his passage through earth-ruled Capricorn. Now we are in the realm of air and ideas, not structures. We can take some calculated risks, especially intellectual ones.

## Meet Uranus, the Modern Planetary Ruler of Aquarius

Uranus is an ice giant and transpersonal planet, discovered in 1781 and thought to be assigned to Aquarius at some point in the nineteenth century, although exactly when is a matter of debate among astrologers. In Greek mythology, Uranus is a sky god associated with the thunderbolt. In astrology, Uranus can help us have breakthroughs and speaks to our rebelliousness. It can snap us out of ruts, sometimes suddenly and shockingly. Connected with technology and mass communication, people with strong Uranus signatures in their charts are often geniuses in these and other realms of abstract ideas.

In my work, Uranus has always made sense as an Aquarian ruler, and this was solidified after Uranus moved into Aquarius from 1995 to 2003. This was when the internet went mainstream, entering many of our homes, and cell phone technology went from obscure to landing in most people's hot little hands. Wi-Fi—literally information beaming through the air, which is maybe the most Aquarian thing EVER—soon followed. Under the tutelage of Saturn, Capricorns learn to remember that their bodies are something of meaning and substance. By the time the Sun passes the torch to airy Aquarius with its shared Uranian rulership, the assignment is to remember that natives *have a body* in the first place.

## Aquarius' Erotic Gifts

There was an alternative weekly in New York City in the late nineties called the *New York Press*. It had all kinds of interesting quirks, but one of my favorite sections to peruse was the personals, where they had all the traditional categories: "Man seeking Woman," "Man seeking Man," etc., and my favorite category, "Whatever's Clever," for everything else.

I think of Aquarians, at their most sexually evolved, as embracers of the concept of "whatever's clever"—they learn what turns them on via experimentation, and may be wide open to kink and all varieties of sextech. Aquarians might just "get" things like virtual reality (VR) sex and advanced teledildonics (electronic or robotic sex toys) before any of their peers, and find themselves introducing the technology to lovers, opening their worlds to what feels truly revolutionary. Their fixed air energy gives them an intellectual focus that can be overwhelmingly cerebral, as if they're always about to have some kind of breakthrough idea that will transform humanity.

Aquarians often keep a collection of friends or chosen family—their beloved freaks and glam geeks (if you haven't seen the brilliant but canceled show *Freaks and Geeks*, go stream it). They may or may not be sleeping with these people, or maybe did in the past, but they're likely to be very good at doing friends-with-benefits arrangements. A powerful Aquarius gift is their ability to identify whatever people may find less socially acceptable about themselves and to accept and love it as it is.

The Aquarian neural network seems interlinked with the entire universe, where conventions no longer exist, and love has always been love. Healthy Aquarians help others to wave their freak flags high, liberating them from prescribed norms and boring conformity. This creates even more space for them to be entirely themselves without worrying about whether their essential self is everyone's cup of tea.

"Compersion" is a poly concept that describes the pleasure experienced when a lover experiences pleasure, even if that pleasure is coming from another lover. Because true friendship seems to be at the core of all Aquarian romantic and sexual relationships, experiencing compersion is less of a stretch for them than others for whom the conventions of love and sex hold sway.

Even if their sexual interests are purely vanilla, Aquarians tend to be open-minded and remain in a place of eternal discovery about their sexuality, recognizing it as an evolutionary force. Sexual liberation, that clarion call of the sixties, is something certain Aquarians can experience and achieve more easily than others. But matching their visionary intellect to the real needs of their bodies—that's where things get complicated.

## Pathway to Play and Creativity for Aquarius

Creativity, lots of it, the weirder the better—this is something Aquarius can usually get it up for. They are highly experimental, and just about any art form is worth trying, just once, to see if it clicks. It's already clear here from the many mentions of sci-fi, but consuming utopian and/or dystopian art or making erotic speculative fiction is something Water Bearers may be pretty adept at, because they can see the future and reflect on the past. Finding a pathway to play that leads to erotic fulfillment might just mean going full tilt into sex tech and gear.

## Aquarius' Erotic Challenges

As open-minded and kink-curious as Aquarians can be when they've done their shadow work, once they find something that turns them on, they may become a bit fixated on it, limiting their continued sexual evolution.

Because Aquarius is a fixed air sign, they can get attached to a particular mental idea about what it is they want and then find that need hard to shake. Aquarians tend to analyze before they can feel into anything, including their desire. Some fetishes, although completely normal, can make it difficult for them to experience pleasure via other outlets. This might be anything from a particular kind of porn to a specific sex toy, position, or recurring fantasy. It should be said: there is nothing wrong with having preferences, knowing what they are, and expressing that to a partner, nor is there anything wrong with going back to what is tried and true. This is only a problem when it stifles an Aquarius, thwarting their ability to move or expand their erotic horizons or connect to a partner intimately. This fetish formation is generally less for sensorial reasons and more because the *idea* of it resonated with them at an early age. The other fixed signs, Taurus (earth), Leo (fire), and Scorpio (water), can grow fixated on sensations, ego, and emotions, respectively. These fixed signs are the hard-core middle children of each of the four seasons, and they tend to get quite stuck in their ways if they don't actively work through it.

Sometimes an early masturbatory fantasy can develop into a fetish, stopping an Aquarius from getting off without it. Fetishes are usually harmless, as long as consent is practiced, but when a fetish becomes the only pathway to sexual desire and expression, it can become problematic for both the fetish-haver and their partner(s).

Additionally, Aquarians can be so caught up in a mental loop that they might forget they even have a body. Like an antenna searching for signals from the universe, they might be attuned to what's "out there" instead of what's going on physically. Calming their hyped-up nervous systems is an essential, if challenging, part of opening up their erotic potential.

## Aquarius Shame and Shadow Work

Being distinctively different and making space for others to follow along is an Aquarian superpower, but being different is also often the source of their shame. Many Aquarians go through a period, often in their tween/teen years, and sometimes even in their twenties or beyond, during which they struggle with being ostracized, or at least feeling like others don't see them. Even Aquarians who are conventionally popular or part of the "in-crowd" tend to secretly feel that they're outside a window looking in while a circle of friends are vibing together. They might respond to this perceived banishment by granting themselves a kind of cool outsider status, playing up the most unconventional things about themselves (through dress or interests), and acting like they don't care about being liked.

This can lead to an inner iciness that mimics Aquarius season weather. It can wall off their heart, numb their gut-brain axis, and make it much harder to tune into pleasure. Yet as detached as they appear, when they are activated by their Leo shadow, they might long to be adored and fawned over. Leos seem to hungrily crave the glow of the spotlight and fall for lovers who are smitten by their charms. Aquarians can heal their shadow when they acknowledge that they secretly desire affection and acceptance from both lover(s) and friends. Rather than redirecting a need to be adored into a broader network of peers, they can become more heart-centered and transform their relationship to love, sex, and human connection—just by melting some of that ice.

Cleo was a forty-seven-year-old Aquarius Sun who identified as nonbinary and was in a polyamorous quad in Brooklyn. The quad had lived together happily for ten years when I met Cleo, who complained of perimenopause symptoms reducing their interest in sex. They felt like they were on the outside looking in at their three partners, who continued to enjoy a robust sex life even as Cleo opted out, feeling like a robotic housemate instead of a lover and romantic partner. We were able to quickly address their physical symptoms with a hyaluronic acid vaginal moisturizer insert, and Cleo hoped this would make the difference, but they returned for another session within a month. Even though they could now comfortably participate in sex with their lovers, they still didn't want to. We had to dig deeper.

Cleo told me a story about coming out as bisexual in college in the early nineties, and how the poor reception they received from friends and family led to tremendous anxiety for which they eventually needed to be medicated. They never fully processed the original trauma of not being accepted by either their straight friends or the queer groups on campus, who at that time were still unwelcoming to bi people. They stopped sharing their identity with new people they met, suffering a major crisis at their Saturn Return. They came out again as nonbinary at thirty-one and finally found their "right tribe." This was a period of major sexual exploration and discovery for Cleo, something they very much wanted to experience again in the present. But they were at the point where even masturbation didn't feel appealing, because, they told me, their entire pelvis felt numb. They admitted that when they first began having libido issues, they felt like their lovers wouldn't accept or feel attracted to them anymore, and it froze them off from their body. Their lovers all came for a session, assuring me they were not rejecting Cleo and that they supported their journey. Yet Cleo's original trauma had been activated and they couldn't turn it off on their own.

I referred Cleo to an EMDR practitioner to process their original coming out trauma, where their progress had been blocked and walled off. They were able to repattern the way they responded to imagined rejection from their lovers, unfreeze their heart, and reconnect to their body, beginning with a self-pleasure routine, then first being with each partner individually to build intimacy, and finally re-experiencing the group sex that they had longed to enjoy again.

When an Aquarian recognizes that they need to do shadow work after realizing something is missing, they must start with finding the places inside that are iced over or numbed out. Figuring out if they've been numb since they first began to experience themselves as a sexual being or somewhere else along the way can make a big difference in their healing process. If the heart itself is walled off because of trauma, practicing being vulnerable may take some time, but it's so worth it to chip away at that ice, bit by bit, until the entire body and soul is warmed up and ready to experience love and passion.

## Journal Questions for Aquarian Shadow Work

- What would happen if I let a lover truly see me?
- Where do I go when I float away?
- How would I describe my future erotic self?
- What if my ideas about pleasure were less rigid?
- What does my heart long for?
- What would happen if I relaxed and felt the joy in every cell of my body?

## A Deeper Look at Body Rulership and Erogenous Zones for Aquarius

Aquarius is the sign of connectivity, and all the regions of the body that connect our systems are under its purview. From the fascial network to the veins and the electrical currents to what we might call the "energetic body," Aquarius is associated with these invisible networks that have their own language. It also rules the ankles, a kind of flexible hinge between our legs and feet.

Turning on an Aquarius body can mean turning on something electric and connective inside of them. This may have nothing to do with the genitals (at least at first) and everything to do with ideas that charge their neural networks and branch out into the rest of their body. This isn't always as simple as taking a hand, kissing the lips, or caressing some other body part (although their sensitive ankles may quickly respond to touch) and may require some experimentation.

Storytelling, fantasy, and kink/fetish exploration using virtual reality simulation can awaken the pleasure centers of an Aquarian body. Trying out all kinds of new sex toys is also a big yes here!

Pre-coital meditation or massage sessions (focusing on the legs, especially the calves, ankles, and shins) can calm Aquarians as it turns them on. It can sometimes be a challenge to soothe an Aquarius nervous system during sex, but tools like this can help them to meet an entirely different side of themselves, and to experience deeper pleasure that opens them up to intimacy with themselves and others.

## An Embodiment Exercise for Aquarius Season

### Erotic Progressive Muscle Relaxation

This practice is based on an exercise originally developed by Dr. Edmund Jacobson. It can be done before solo or partnered sex or just for the purpose of relaxation before sleep.

Lie down in bed or on the floor. Close your eyes if you feel comfortable and take five deep, slow breaths into your belly, with exhales longer than inhales. Bring your awareness to your genital region or any other part of the body that you associate with being turned on. As you move through the different muscle groups, bring your awareness back to this part of the body and observe how it changes, relaxes, or activates.

Begin with the feet—lift your toes upward, hold for three seconds, then point them downward and hold for three seconds. Release. Notice how your ankles feel. Now move to your calves, tensing them for three seconds, then release. Draw your knees together for three seconds, then release. Now move to your thighs, tense them for three seconds, then release.

Bring your awareness to your genital area and clench your perineum, as if you're doing a Kegel, hold for three seconds, and release. Now hold your belly tense for three seconds, and release. Now tense your hands, hold for three seconds, and release. Now contract your arms, hold for three seconds, and release.

Now take a deep inhale and hold it for three seconds, releasing in an exhale for a bit longer. Raise your shoulders, hold for three seconds, and release. Purse your lips, hold for three seconds, and release. Open your mouth wide for three seconds, then release and close it. Open your eyes for three seconds, then close them to release. Now lift your eyebrows, hold for three seconds, then release.

Return your awareness to the part of your body you originally designated as your "turn on" area, whether it's the genitals or some other part of you. Imagine pink light emanating from this area to the rest of your body, up, down, and around, like you're bathing yourself in the energy of desire. Take a few more deep breaths into this part of your body. If you feel like pleasuring yourself, go right ahead.

## Try These Tools to Connect to Aquarius Energy:

- Explore using electro-stim sex toys.
- Go to a cuddle party.
- Take a breath orgasm workshop.
- Think yourself off (Google it!).
- Practice grounding exercises like taking a weighted nature walk.
- Offer community care and accept it when it is offered to you.

# 13

# Pisces Sexuality

## Merging and Mysticism

I was in love with the whole world and all that lived in its rainy arms.

**Louise Erdrich**

*Love Medicine*

**Dates:** February 19–March 21

**Sexual Archetype:** The Spiritual Awakener

**Motivation:** Compassion

**Symbol:** The Fish

**Planetary Ruler:** Jupiter (Traditional, also rules Sagittarius) and Neptune (Modern)

**Element:** Water

**Modality:** Mutable

**Erogenous Zones and Body Rulership:** The Feet and Lymphatic System

Healthy Pisces energy is dreamy, magical, sensitive, imaginative, fantastical, glamorous, oceanic, luminescent, empathetic, and totally transcendent. The Fish shimmers in the ocean's depths, revealing an infinite number of iridescent possibilities. All of consciousness is here, uncontained. Pisces can take the body beyond the body, tuning into cosmic messages that most mere mortals miss.

Profound sexual healing of self and other is within reach when Pisces tunes into its own inner depths, but when this sign becomes overwhelmed by the world and its discontents, it can drown in escapism. Here, pleasure is numbed and true intimacy grows exhausting. If a Pisces can keep their delicate feet planted firmly on the ground while channeling healing messages from the universe, pleasure can be utterly rapturous and continuous, as if all of life is bathed in orgasm.

Yes, I know that sounds a little out there—but that's the point with Pisces. It's a sign and a feeling that's not quite of this Earth. For Pisces, it can feel challenging just to exist in a body. This is one of the reasons they tend to love sleep—and often really enjoy getting high.

## Dream On: Pisces Season in Focus

Here we are at the end of the zodiacal wheel, where we become one with the beginning again. In Pisces season in the Northern Hemisphere, the big freeze may still be on at the start, but we know we can at least *hope* to go out like a lamb later in March. *Hope* is such a Pisces word, evoking the promise of renewal to come if we're willing to go as deep as we can in the moment. As we leave Aquarius season for Pisces season, we're moving from thinking to feeling. Because it's hard to know in advance if we'll catch a wintry squall or the promise of a spring-like day when we can loosen our coats and feel the warmth on our faces, tuning into the accompanying emotional swell helps us orient ourselves in time and space.

Pisces season steeps us in mutable water that flows. In Cancer season, the water moodily and cyclically crashes against the shore. In Scorpio season it is contained, either in a cauldron simmering to a boil or possibly in an ice cube. By the time we get to Pisces season, we are the entire body of water, a universe unto itself, boundless and beckoning us to dive down to the depths of the past, present, and all possible sexual futures. We have exited the quantum time of Aquarius season and entered a lucid dream space: our psyches are ripe for healing.

We may be more erotically intuitive now. Lovemaking can feel like soul-merging, even in casual encounters. When we give ourselves orgasms, the moment of release might transport us to a place we've never been. Our dreams may be psychic and lucid—perhaps we'll connect to a lover we've lost and missed, and when we wake up, we feel like we spent authentic time with them on a different plane.

Our sensitivity may be heightened now, making us receptive to desires and attractions we may not have picked up on in more abstract, intellectual astrological seasons, especially the just completed Aquarius season. Pisces season often feels like a palliative to this recent season of the mind. If Aquarius connected us to our community, Pisces season can connect us to the entire cosmos. Now we might ask the question: What does the universe want me to know about my desire? We may not receive answers that speak to traditional ways of "knowing"—we're better off tuning into the signs all around us.

## Get to Know Jupiter (Again), the Traditional Planetary Ruler of Pisces

In Sagittarius, Jupiter is a born adventurer in search of worldly wisdom, boldly going to places where others may not dare to roam. In Pisces, Jupiter takes us to all corners of the sea, expanding exponentially in waves of oceanic enormity. Here Jupiter's essential desire—to know—is sated only by an immersion in the collective unconscious. This is not the kind of knowledge you can get through books or even cultural experiences or religious teachings. This is the kind of knowingness you can get only by plugging into everything that has ever been and everything that's still to come by accessing your intuition. That place where we already know the answers to all our questions—that's where Jupiter moves as the ruler of Pisces. Jupiter wanders around looking for external truth as Sagittarius' ruler, but in Pisces, it searches for the universal truth within.

## Meet Neptune, the Modern
## Planetary Ruler of Pisces

I like to call Neptune "the planet of pink fog." Not a big fan of the harsh light of reality, Neptune is a dream weaver, escape artist, and magic maker all rolled into one transpersonal planet. At its highest vibration, Neptune is deeply creative and healing. At the lower vibration, Neptune can be deceptive and misleading, like a pretty mist concealing a foreboding city. Sometimes Neptune makes us feel like we're in a swirl of "delulu" energy, that perfectly apt colloquialism derived from the word "delusion" and born during the Neptune-in-Pisces age. Neptune can immerse a person in deception and slippery snake-oil salesmanship during harsher transits, but Neptune is also where Pisces gets its spiritual glamour.

## Pisces' Erotic Gifts

As the sign that feels *everything*, Pisces can experience the most extraordinary, exquisite erotic highs. Fishes can feel every vibe, every nuance of emotion, every single sensation, long before anyone has touched them, sometimes even before a word is whispered, a call is made, or a text is sent by a lover. Sometimes their solo sex sessions are preceded by the psychic sense that someone they love (or once loved) is thinking about them or "calling" them through the ether. Pisces have been known to dial up lovers erotically and psychically just by using them for fantasy fodder, too. Pisces' facility for fantasy rivals all other signs. They can imagine intricate scenarios and dream them into existence. This is a learned skill for many, but for Fishes, it often comes quite naturally, and fantasies sometimes feel so real that they can sustain an erotic high that goes on for days or weeks, solo or shared. These elaborate, large-scale, Hollywood-style fantasies can also fuel partnered sex and role-playing situations, if they have a willing playmate.

Pisces eroticism is often about the urge to merge; Fishes may long to find a soul connection, even for just one night. For Pisces, connecting at a spiritual level that makes space for leaving bodies behind can be a big plus. There can be a need to wash the world away—with all of its fear, pain, trauma, and worry. Giving this compassion to a partner erotically can up the ante for Pisces, increasing their own pleasure. Pisces is one of the signs that truly, madly, and deeply gets off on feeling a lover get off.

Even though they live in human bodies, it's important to understand that Pisces often aren't *of* their bodies. They might seem transcendent, floating above and beyond mundane notions of physiology and sexual mechanics. Sexual intuition is another Piscean asset. With lovers, they can anticipate what should come next, sometimes even before their partner knows how to name their own desire. We've established that Pisces can experience an unrivaled and purely energetic eroticism. And because they tend to be extremely sensitive in all ways, including physically, they can melt into a kind of orgasmic pool from the lightest touch. Because of this, the sex they have can be simple in mechanics, straightforward and vanilla, and yet make it seem as if pink, glittery manna is pouring down from the heavens.

## Pathway to Play and Creativity for Pisces

Pisces rules the feet, and although this sign is connected to all art forms, dance can feel like an exquisite emotional release, both watching others dance and moving their own bodies. This is often a big turn-on for Pisces people, and dancing before sex, solo or partnered, is a deeply soulful and highly erotic experience for them. Pisces can also experience creative ecstasy through Tarot pulls, meditation, writing or reading poetry, honing their psychic skillset, keeping a dream journal, and having deeper than deep, nonlinear conversations with beloveds who honor their need to emote.

## Pisces' Erotic Challenges

Pisces' renowned compassion is a gift, but they must work hard to learn how to construct and maintain healthy boundaries or else they can drown in other people's problems. Lovers often assume they possess an endless well of empathy that magically refreshes itself like an enchanted spring and end up taking advantage of that. Often a Pisces will give and give and give, especially to lovers, until their own well runs dry. This depletion of resources can also exhaust their erotic capacities.

Day-to-day reality can also erode the Piscean urge to feel desire. In many ways they need to weave or witness the weaving of magic to experience an erotic charge. In sexual relationships, once that magical veneer begins to fade, a normal thing that happens in relationships over time, a Pisces may look for escape hatches. They need regular sprinklings of fresh pixie dust to access that erotic longing again.

The old "put on your own oxygen mask first" adage is an important one for Pisces, especially when they sense their sexual desire is evaporating. Sometimes a Pisces feels like they might die without a connection to a beloved, past or present. They have to be reminded that love is everywhere, all the time, and even if they don't currently have the Big Love that fuels their imagination and fantasy life, they can create that intimacy in their relationship with their own body.

Some Pisces become saviors in order to defend against their need to be rescued, pushing themselves to protect and shield every human and animal they meet, all to prevent themselves from feeling unsafe. They might then blame a lover for failing them before they've had a chance to show they care. Wounds from early childhood can translate to addictions as an adult, and although I don't use the term "sex addiction" (because I don't believe we can be addicted to a process that is a basic human need, as discussed earlier), Pisces can sometimes act out sexually with multiple partners even when they're not genuinely interested in experimenting with ethical non-monogamy. This tends to happen when they feel traumatized, unsupported, and disconnected from their souls.

An exceptionally sensitive young Pisces can certainly turn to various addictions to blunt their traumas or the traumas they've absorbed from their loved ones. They need to guard against developing a victim/martyr complex or codependent patterns in their sexual relationships and find ways to tune into their own pleasure daily—not just spiritually, but physically. Developing healthy, safe, enriching outlets for their escapist drive can be grounding. This might be meditation, art making, or somatic therapy.

## Pisces Shame and Shadow Work

The extreme sensitivity of living in a Pisces body is incomparable to any other astrological experience. For those who lack any Pisces planets, it can be hard to understand intellectually—in the same way reading or watching a movie about space travel isn't going to make you feel what astronauts *feel* when they ascend above the Earth and view their tiny blue home planet from the expanse. Pisces are all feeling, all the time. This is overwhelming, and the tendency can be to tune out of this emotional sphere simply to escape the barrage of their own empathy. Because they're constantly swimming through the deep waters of their psyche, in some ways, Pisces are always plunging into a kind of shadow work—it's just deeply disorganized. Pisces tend to carry deep shame about their inner "mess," often feeling like a failure when they can't control their emotions. When they fall in love hard, fast, and instantly, then have what feels like magical, soul-sustaining sex with a partner, time can stop briefly. But when the physical connection ends, because their partner needs to get up to go to the bathroom or take a call—the vagaries of reality—the Pisces soul can feel wholly eviscerated. All they want is to merge, and when they realize they are back in their singular body again, it can feel like they're alone and drowning.

When Jennifer, a cishet woman in her late forties, booked a session with me, her email began with: "HELP! I'm a love addict and I can't stop making bad decisions about sex." She had the Sun, Venus, and Moon in Pisces, and they were all being activated by a Neptune transit when she reached out to me. A nurse, recently divorced with three kids, she had lived through a mostly sexless marriage, taking care of everyone, including her husband, who was more like her child than her partner. When she did have sex with him, she found herself so concerned about his release that she disassociated and couldn't feel her own body. She had spent the years since her divorce trying to find her erotic spark again and kept ending up hurt and unsatisfied. But she was more focused on the emotional hurt than the pleasure deficit.

She carried a lot of shame around the idea that she was too emotional, having been told to rein in her big feelings by everyone from her mother, as a child, to all of her boyfriends and eventually, by her ex-husband. She often used the word "mess" to describe her feelings and her life. The more she thought of herself this way, the more she felt like she couldn't live without a glass of wine at dinner, which turned into two glasses, and sometimes more after her kids went to bed.

In our work together, we first addressed the roots of that shame and the ways families, partners, and a culture of toxic masculinity diminish the primacy of emotional expression. She began to realize that the people in her life who shamed her for her feelings were just looking for ways not to deal with their own. The world is not always friendly to empathic Pisces people, and we began to reframe her sensitivity as a superpower, rather than a form of self-sabotage.

When I asked what genuine erotic pleasure might be for her, her first response was, "A loving partner who will help me." So I asked: "What would genuine erotic pleasure be for you *in your body*?" She had spent so many years serving others without focusing on her own pleasure that she could no longer remember what felt good. She wondered if she ever knew.

I gave her home-play exercises that required finding time alone without any responsibilities lingering outside her bedroom door. We agreed that taking a bath every evening was the best way for her to get privacy and make time for pleasure. She bought a waterproof clitoral vibrator, and every night for two weeks she gave herself an orgasm and meditated afterward, spending at least a half hour in the tub. I told her to alternate between fantasizing about whatever came to mind and simply using the toy with her eyes closed, just focusing on the sensation in her genitals until orgasm, imagining the orgasmic energy flooding around her body in the form of pink light, reaching to each of her limbs and encircling her, creating an imaginary boundary of pleasure and self-love. This practice radically transformed Jennifer's relationship to pleasure and her body. When she embarked on a new relationship, she was able to clearly communicate her needs—emotional, sexual, and practical—without feeling like she was risking rejection.

Taking a note from their opposite sign, Virgo, can help Pisces to navigate the chaotic expanse of their beautiful psyches with a compass and a map instead of merely floating in whatever direction the tides are moving at any given time. This might mean doing directed dream work in a more careful, calculated way, perhaps with the input of a Jungian therapist or another practitioner who works with symbols.

If that's not possible, rather than waking up and briefly considering a dream image or posting "I had the weirdest dream" on social media, keeping a dedicated dream journal on their nightstand and writing an entry each morning (or recording it to a specific file on their phone) can help to reorient all those feelings and make more logical sense of how, why, and when they float to the surface of their subconscious. This is not to control their feelings but to avoid drowning in them.

## Journal Questions for Pisces Shadow Work

- Am I afraid of my reality? Why?

- What would happen if I drew firmer boundaries with a lover, past, present, or future?

- What does my soul desire in explicit, erotic terms?

- How can I make my fantasies real?

- What do I want to dream about tonight?

## A Deeper Look at Body Rulership and Erogenous Zones for Pisces

Pisces rules the feet, and their own tend to be quite sensitive to both pleasure and problems. Paying extra attention to the feet for grounding, healing, and releasing sensation should be on regular rotation for people who live in Pisces bodies. Foot massage, tickling, toe sucking, and foot jobs (when the genitals are stimulated by a foot) can really turn on a Fish. Fishes may try to play footsie under the table at dinner as a fun kind of foreplay.

Taking care of the feet for health and aesthetic reasons is highly recommended. This might mean investing in monthly pedicures regardless of gender (or doing them at home with a kit), considering a once-yearly medical pedicure, and incorporating holistic foot care like reflexology and simple foot rolling, using a yoga ball.

Even more than their sister water signs Cancer and Scorpio, Pisces tend to enjoy being immersed in bodies of water. From flotation tanks to a warm tub with a few drops of an aphrodisiac essential oil, Fishes can relax deeply when immersed in their sign's element. Sexy romps in the sea, hot tub, or bathtub are also ways to get a Fish's libido flowing.

## An Embodiment Exercise for Pisces Season

### Visualizing Pleasure

You can do this exercise anytime you need to feel grounded; it's especially potent before partnered or solo sex, to remind you how to be in your body and feel all the sensations. It can be done almost anywhere, but may feel soothing in a bath, shower, or in or near a body of water (on the beach, at the edge of a lake, etc.).

Whatever position feels comfortable is fine—if you're someplace you can lie down comfortably or float, that's great, but sitting in a chair works too. Close your eyes if you feel comfortable and take three or four long, deep breaths into your pelvis (your second or sacral chakra), holding for a moment and releasing stress, self-blame, and shame in the breath as it moves upward along the spine, exhaling through the top of your head (your seventh or crown chakra). As you let out each breath, you can either say out loud or silently say to yourself what (or who) you're releasing. Perhaps it's an old lover's name, an unhealthy habit, or an unsatisfying sex life.

On your next inhale, imagine a pale green light hovering above your head and then visualize it drawing through your crown chakra like a mist, over your head and face, neck and shoulders, down your spine, hovering for an extra moment around any parts of your body that need healing, then over your pelvis and down and around your legs until it gets to your feet. As the light travels down, in and around your body, it forms a kind of sheath or bubble, encircling you in a safe, beautiful place where your boundaries cannot be crossed. Now the light begins to glow even brighter, as it encircles the tops of your feet and toes and soles and spends a few moments there, healing, restoring, and giving love to this part of your body.

With your body and spirit completely encircled in this bright, soothing, mystical green light, visualize what you would want your body to do and be if you didn't have to caretake anyone else. What pleasure would you give yourself? A delicious meal from your favorite restaurant? A night in a five-star hotel where you could have sex with a doting lover all day and night? Or time with your favorite sex toy that no responsibility can infringe upon? Imagine this in glorious Technicolor detail. Spend as much time as you want here in this special fantasy place. When you're done, see the green light slowly evaporate, as if the sheet of mist is gently disappearing, like a genie being revealed. Before completely disappearing, the light gathers at your feet and transforms into a ball. Imagine this ball rising to your heart and entering your body, where it will stay with you forever, protecting you and offering you the pleasure that you deserve any time—on demand.

## Try These Tools to Connect with Pisces Energy:

- Keep an erotic dream journal.

- Get regular pedicures, with an extra ten-minute foot massage. Give them to yourself, or let a lover attend to your toes.

- Walk on the earth without shoes as often as possible and try grounding or earthing exercises.

- Take dance classes! Or just put on your favorite playlist and dance when you feel stressed or want to awaken your libido.

- Try walking meditation or other active kinds of contemplative practices.

# 14

## Venus

### The Pleasure of Receiving

Beauty is truth, truth beauty.

**John Keats**

"Ode on a Grecian Urn"


I want your hands on me.

**Sinead O'Connor**

*The Lion and the Cobra*


**Names of Venus in Other Cultures:** Sumerian:
Inanna; Babylonian: Ishtar; Egyptian: Isis; Greek:
Aphrodite; Norse: Freya; Indian: Parvati

**Venus Rules:** the earth sign Taurus and
the air sign Libra

**Flower:** The Rose

**Day of the Week:** Friday

**Keywords:** beauty, love, desire, sex, connection,
art, relational energy, sensuality, pleasure, hedonism,
partnership, intimacy, creativity, refinement, sociability

Venus has many appellations and has appeared in myriad cultures over the millennia. To deepen our understanding of the astrology of sexuality, in this book we're working with a planetary derivation of the Roman version of Venus, the goddess of love and beauty. Venus, in essence, shows us how to define and deify what is beautiful, worthy, inviting, erotic, romantic, desirable, and lovable about ourselves—she lays out our offerings, showing us the ways that our pleasure expands in the act of receiving, and fundamentally, how we desire to be received by others.

Venus lives in the realms of the sensual as a ruler of Taurus, and the socially acceptable, aesthetically pleasing, and artful, as a ruler of Libra. There is a bit of a split here in the Venusian personality—she seesaws between the wild and the rational. The brilliant late astrologer Erin Sullivan dives into this in her wonderful book *Venus and Jupiter: Bridging the Ideal and the Real*. But no matter what sign your own natal Venus is in (I delve into each unique Venus sign later in the chapter), this planet can show you much about the way you love and want to be loved. When Venus is prominent in our natal chart or when our personal Venus is elicited by a transit or an erotic experience, the response may come from the wild Venus or the rational Venus, or somewhere in between.

The Latin word *Venus* is derived from the roots of the Proto-Indo-European word for desire. And indeed, Venus can show us how *we want to be wanted*. This is an often-unexplored arena in sexuality—how do we understand the parts of ourselves that *create desire* through the act and the art of *being desired*? What comes first, the wanting or the being wanted?

Desire, defined by verb forms *to want, to crave, to covet*—this is our body and mind responding to what we see, smell, touch, taste, or hear. This can happen in an instant—in what we might call love at first sight—or over time, as we develop desire by getting to know someone and building intimacy. We can project our desires onto a crush who doesn't know us at all, onto a cute barista or colleague or classmate or celebrity or influencer with whom we form a parasocial relationship. When this happens, our Venus is there, showing us what our erotic taste is.

Yet, it's much more complicated than that, because Venus also shows us the kind of lover we are, feel ourselves to be, or perhaps the one we hope to be. Our natal Venus can describe the way we dress or wear our hair, our favorite perfume, the way we flirt, how we show up for a lover, how we make love, and where that may lead to.

Getting to the higher octaves of any Venus placement may first require an interrogation—not of what seduces us, but how we think we're *meant to seduce others*. Once we work through these expectations, we can get back to the essentials of the erotic nature of Venus, and properly explore her sensual potentials.

## How Venus Bears Gifts and Shadows

Venus, as the Lesser Benefic to Jupiter's Greater Benefic designation, often comes in light and sweet. It's not that she's superficial, but she tends to provide us with ease, often in the guise of beauty and sensuality. Desire, worship, and love are her gifts. Benefics ostensibly bring us joy. Don't worry that Venus is known as "lesser"; it may be because she's a smaller planet with a shorter orbit, and that the joys she delivers are intimate and personal, where Jupiter's joys are sweeping and boundless. When a little bit of well-directed Venusian joy hits us in the right spot at the right time, it can have a lasting impact on the way we feel about ourselves. We might even call that our "V-spot."

Like every planet in our chart, Venus has a shadow, and acknowledging this is central to having a healthy, thriving, and pleasurable call-and-response with your own natal Venus placement. One quick way to assess the shadow of our Venus placement is to look at its opposite sign and see what we may be denying or shutting down about our erotic nature. Rather than name that as "not me!" we might try to explore and experiment with it a bit.

Our natal Venus wants us to experience pleasure in a particular way, and if we keep having romantic, relational, or purely sexual experiences that leave us disappointed, confused, and/or wanting more, we might look to the shadow of our natal Venus to see what we may be enacting. When Venus shows up as shadow, she often comes in as jealousy, low self-esteem (especially in terms of how attractive we feel), and sometimes as excess.

To understand how Venus comes through in our charts and our lives, it also helps to look at her workings along with her partner-in-crime, Mars, the planet of passion and the action star of the next chapter. Astrologers call Venus and Mars lovers or cosmic consorts. In the simplest terms, devoid of human gender identities or sexual preferences, Venus receives, and Mars pushes and probes. Venus opens and welcomes, while Mars extends and defends. Venus beckons, while Mars thrusts. Venus relaxes and calms, while Mars activates and excites. When these two planets are well-aspected in a natal chart or in synastry or compatibility charts (the charts of two or more people in relationship to one another), sparks of attraction often fly.

## Working with Transiting Venus

The Greeks knew our Venus by two names: Phosphorus when she appeared as a morning star, and Hesperus when she appeared as an evening star. When the Romans named the planet Venus, it was in part because its resplendent beauty evoked their goddess Venus, who was drawn from the Greek Aphrodite. Venus, the bestower of love, beauty, and desire, was given to a planet with an orbit that reminded them of the perfect petals of a rose (more on that in a bit). They knew nothing about the surface of the planet Venus (a thick, toxic atmosphere of carbon dioxide and sulfuric acid) or that it is the hottest planet in the solar system.

Despite all of this, Venus is the closest and most similar planet to Earth. She's like family, a sibling in the sky reminding us of home. Arguably the most beautiful planet to gaze at with the naked eye, her bright light is impossible not to notice, like a flirtatious potential lover beckoning us into their orbit. From our perspective, Venus is never more than forty-seven degrees away from the Sun, keeping her always luminous and inviting. No wonder the Romans first thought of their love goddess Venus when they chose her assignation.

Venus appears to us either as a morning star or an evening star—we might say she has two faces in this way—as well as in her Taurus/

Libra split. Many traditions ascribe militarist qualities to the morning star version of Venus. In fact, all astrological traditions except for (modern) Western astrology and Vedic astrology include both versions of Venus—the lover and the warrior.

## Venus, Beauty Myths, and Patriarchy

Let's further probe the concept of how often *we want to be wanted* when it comes to love and sex. For all the sweet complexities inherent in a discussion of Venus, especially for those of us who identify as intersectional feminists, there is something fundamental about looking at Venus through the lens of how we expect to be received by society because of what we've internalized about beauty standards. I find that working through this before engaging with some of the typical assignations of Venus through the signs in our chart is essential and profound, even for cishet men.

Patriarchy has toxified and negatively flavored our perceptions of our bodies and vilified sensuality for most who don't live in bodies that are white and male—to me this is a given and the process of undoing that bullshit is ongoing. I've been working on this my entire life, often through my relationship with my own body and through my natal Venus in Pisces. But even for those with the most privilege—the aforementioned white and male-bodied amongst us—there are myriad, pernicious body image issues that often exist alongside and are intertwined with sexual functioning issues. Part of grappling with these twisted cultural expectations means we must integrate and understand how Venus shows up in shadow in order to live with more freedom and authenticity. Venus, at her best in our charts, shows us how we can experience the heights of erotic pleasure, but first we must work through the baggage patriarchy loads her down with.

John Berger's art criticism book *Ways of Seeing* framed the male gaze, simply, as "men act, and women appear." We can substitute all marginalized bodies for "women" here when we say that LGBTQIA+ bodies, Black and brown and indigenous bodies, and all bodies under a system of structuralized racism and heteropatriarchy are not meant to consume, but are meant *to be consumed* by the dominant culture. Unpacking this as we examine the intricacies of our own natal Venus placement, its aspects to other planets, how we experience it in transit, and how it "plays with others" in synastry can provide us with a much deeper dive into our own desire nature.

## A Quick Overview of Venus in Your Chart

You can easily find your natal Venus placement using free astrology apps or astro.com, which is perhaps the quickest and easiest, but even if you've read descriptions of your natal Venus placement elsewhere, you can use these descriptions as a lens into the way your Venus sign wants to be wanted and how it may find pleasure in receiving.

### Venus in Aries

Venus is in detriment in Aries as the opposite sign to Libra where she is in domicile. (*Detriment*, in short, is when a planet doesn't feel super comfortable in a particular sign and has to work a little harder to express itself. When planets are in domicile, it means that they're contentedly hanging out in the sign that they rule.) In Aries, Venus can have trouble expressing herself socially, especially in the charts of people whose genders are marginalized. This Venus is naturally assertive and tends to understand more easily what it wants when it sees (or smells) what it wants. It may desire more aggressive touch or "manhandling" by a partner, or more friction during solo sex. Once this Venus pushes through shadow concerns about appearing overly pushy or insistently flirtatious, it can thrive. Different than some of the meeker Venus placements, Venus in Aries can more easily own and transform wanting to be wanted and turn it into its own brand of active desire.

### Venus in Taurus

Venus rules Taurus, making her at home here, allowing those with this placement to feel more relaxed and content in their bodies and around other bodies. There can be an essential comfort around embracing deep sensuality that rarely goes unnoticed. Expressing desire through the five senses naturally and contentedly, like a cat hanging out in a sunbeam without a care in the world—this Venus embodies that vibe. They want to be wanted as if they want to be devoured by touch, taste, sight, smell, and hearing. The Venus in Taurus shadow can feel guilt about overindulgence, gluttony, and laziness, not as a problem in itself, but more as a barrier to feeling like they are lovable.

## Venus in Gemini

This Venus receives pleasure from teaching, learning, and communicating information. It excels at the art of flirtation, and the quicker the wit, the hotter the exchange. Venus in Gemini can make others feel smart because of its fast verbal pace, and it wants very much to receive feedback about its intelligence. This Venus may want to be told (using all manner of mediums from text to talk to emojis) how much it is loved and appreciated. Verbal affection is the elixir of Venus in Gemini desire. The shadow here is excessive flattery—this Venus might go on and on about how amazing a lover is, because they are craving that validation themselves.

## Venus in Cancer

Venus in Cancer craves absolute devotion, and gets intense pleasure out of caring for, comforting, and offering security to partners. This Venus wants to receive physical feedback that evokes the sensation that they will never be left alone. Being enfolded, hugged, held, cuddled—these can all be deeply erotic for Venus in Cancer. The need to feel safe can cause them to hold in their desires for a long period of time, making them seem even more ardent when they do, eventually, allow themselves to touch and be touched. The Venus in Cancer shadow can be overbearing, smothering, and codependent to the extreme. Creating erotic comfort that is not based on emotional dependency is key.

## Venus in Leo

Venus in Leo craves praise and adulation, often giving others the lavish loving that it wants to receive. We might think of this like a cat demanding to be petted. Royally appointed surroundings and decadent courting can increase erotic responsiveness with this Venus. Once this champagne bottle is uncorked, passion spills over with unflagging creativity, enthusiasm, and stamina, but if worship from a lover appears to flag, Venus in Leo can grow quickly bored and even dramatically despondent. Their shadow is jealousy and the provocation of jealousy—the idea that they might go unseen can cause them to act out.

## Venus in Virgo

Venus is in its fall in Virgo, as the opposite of Pisces, where the love goddess exalts. Pleasure for this Venus requires relaxation and deactivation of hypervigilance. This Venus often must work a little harder to receive erotic feedback, as its natural state can engender worry about whether they are attractive and lovable. Stress dampens libido faster than any factor, and Venus in Virgo can find itself neurotically nitpicking lovers and potential lovers instead of trying to figure out what feels good. Pleasure can be found in the details: knowing their bodies well through solo sex practice and the willingness to share this with lovers explicitly. The Venus in Virgo shadow can be criticism when a lover is imperfect, sexually, domestically, or in other ways.

## Venus in Libra

Venus is in domicile in Libra as in Taurus, making the love planet feel mostly groovy and comfortable in this sign. In Libra territory, Venus takes adornment very seriously and aesthetics go hand-in-hand with both sex and the sensation of sexiness. Pleasure can be derived from waiting, slow seduction, and a courtship with all the pretty trimmings. They know how to receive admiration, and they seem to be quite used to it, but their shadow reveals how they're afraid to be alone, without a partner on their arm. Bonding with a lover can be quite stunningly beautiful, but does it reach to the deep places? Another shadow of Venus in Libra is superficiality. People with this placement are better off when they confront and activate their erotic hunting instinct on a regular basis and take the leash off their animal instincts.

## Venus in Scorpio

Venus in Scorpio is, just like Aries, in detriment because it is opposite Taurus where Venus is in domicile. But this Venus still has plenty to work with when it comes to receiving pleasure. This Venus wants to be wanted completely, ultimately, without reservation. There is rarely moderation here—erotic intensity tends to rule. It wants to be consumed by a lover, not merely seduced. Venus in Scorpio can create a shadow that fears expressing love or lust, as it can expose a soft underbelly of emotional vulnerability that can only be soothed by cutting off, ghosting, or leaving a lover to protect their own heart. If these fears are faced rationally and explored, Venus in Scorpio can experience exultant and continuous pleasure.

## Venus in Sagittarius

Venus in Sagittarius wants to be wanted as an adventurer. This Venus feels seen by a lover who recognizes their innate wisdom and insight along with their awkwardness, and would be happy to spend an entire night talking about religion, philosophy, or comedy as a foreplay. They long to be received as fiercely independent, curious, and devil-may-care. There can be immense pleasure in embracing sexual shenanigans— eroticism that is just plain fun. The Venus in Sagittarius shadow is commitment. Even when they fall in love, if they haven't worked out the higher meaning of a sexual connection, they may charge away like a wild horse, finding something else on the horizon.

## Venus in Capricorn

Venus in Capricorn often wants to be received as powerful and in control. This can be a deliciously sensual Venus placement, one that likes to take its time. Yet access to that sensuality may be lacking until the native engages with their desire for power and explores any shadow material around it. Sometimes this Venus will caretake a lover almost relentlessly, refusing any comfort in return (but quietly longing for it). They may find deep erotic release in BDSM practices, either in the dominant, submissive, or switch role (a switch is someone who can go back and forth between dom and sub roles).

## Venus in Aquarius

This Venus receives pleasure via intellectual stimulation, and feels seen and valued when lovers recognize their weirder tendencies, especially when seeing this makes them more interested in engaging erotically. Once these quirks are validated and embraced, they can provide immense pleasure, especially when shared. The shadow here is societal—Venus in Aquarius can have turn-ons and tastes that are considered kinky, and they may struggle with this until getting validation from a peer group, lover, or lovers.

## Venus in Pisces

Venus is exalted in Pisces—best positioned to receive all the love planet's many gifts. This Venus longs to spiritually connect to a lover, and can experience an almost religious fervor when it comes to emotionally connected, intuitive sex. It wants to be received as a force for erotic healing, yet can have trouble communicating in words about what their bodies long for. If they project too much of their own healing spirit onto a lover or lovers, they can fixate on that love object for years, even waiting for them and not giving themselves pleasure, because, they believe, why cheat on God? This Venus must know that they, themselves, are the deity they've been waiting for.

## Managing Transits to the Natal Venus

Once we understand more about our natal Venus, or the sign Venus was in when we were born, we can begin to look at how Venus interacts with other planets to deepen our erotic self-knowledge, and to use these movements to track the way our desires, erotic development, and sexuality evolve over time.

What is a transit? After we're born, the planets keep on moving, and every time one of those planets creates a mathematical angle to one of our own natal/birth chart placements or moves through a house of our charts, we say that planet is "transiting" there—moving from place to place.

Libra and Taurus risings may feel Venus transits the most, as Venus is their chart ruler. If this is you, or your natal Venus is exalted (that's you, Venus in Pisces people), or if you have any personal planet place-ments (the Moon, Mercury, Mars, Jupiter, or Saturn) in the Venus-ruled signs, you might want to pay special attention to Venus as she moves through the zodiac, changing signs every three to four weeks, except during Venus Retrograde phases when she spends a *long* time in one or two signs. I delve into this more in the next section.

We feel transits to our natal Venus the most when outer or transper-sonal planets make "harder" angles to it. Softer angles are always nice! But I want us to work with our challenges to evoke our erotic power, so we'll focus on the rougher stuff, from the outside in. So below, I am describing squares, oppositions, and conjunctions to our natal Venus. I am including Mars and Venus transits in this section, even though they are personal planets, because of their relevance and their relationship to each other.

A whole slew of free apps and websites can tell you when you're hav-ing these transits. I like astro.com (free with paid options), astro-seek.com (great for those who are into traditional astrology), and the TimePassages and Astro Gold apps (free with paid upgrade features, easy-to-use, and comprehensive).

Here are some of the experiences that can be elicited during a hard transit to your natal Venus, depending on the planet involved.

## Pluto

A powerful personal erotic regeneration can take place over a long period of time. Our love and sex lives may be entirely turned inside out, as if we're churned to dust and reborn in a cleansing fire of desire. Opening ourselves up to the transformation is the best way to endure it.

## Neptune

Holy projection, Batman! Neptune transits to the natal Venus can open us to an empathy so vast that we completely lose sight of our own bound-aries. This transit can create illusions that feel glittery and magical, but also delusions that sink us to the bottom of our own proverbial deep sea. Neptune has a dissolving effect, and by the end of this long-term transit, we may feel like part of our erotic self has been washed away. Under Neptune transits we may see the best in our lovers, but by the end, once that illusion is shattered, we might just realize their erotic power was part of us all along.

## Uranus

Sudden alterations to our experience of desire can arrive without warning under a Uranus transit to our natal Venus. This can come as a complete shock to us and our partners. Sometimes this is a new lover showing up who reveals a side of ourselves we never experienced before, but sometimes it's running into a book, movie, culture, sex toy, or some other unexpected encounter that rocks our erotic world.

## Saturn

As the Big Daddy and boundary maker of the heavens, Saturn likes to teach us lessons. When he comes into contact with our natal Venus, we can experience a sense of lack, loneliness, or drought in our love and sex lives, no matter our relationship status. Saturn on our Venus tries to teach us how to slow down and build healthy, safe, long-term scaffolding around our sexual selfhood. Even if it feels boring or challenging, this year-long transit can help us for the long haul.

## Jupiter

Even if it's a transit with a harder edge, it's hard not to love it when the Greater Benefic meets the Lesser Benefic. Jupiter transits to our natal Venus can turn the pleasure in our lives on LOUD. Planning dates, vacations, masturbation marathons, sexy shopping trips—all of these can be extra sweet when Jupiter offers Venus a chance to expand.

## Mars

It's getting hot in here! When Mars hits our natal Venus, it can feel like the Jiffy Lube of libido tune-ups. This is a very horny transit, and it can feel like it's come straight out of the blue if we haven't been paying attention to our chart. It can make us feel a kind of unexpected animal attraction to people we never thought of as potential lovers, and create a kind of itch that can't be scratched without an orgasm, whether given to ourselves or provided by someone else.

## Venus

When transiting Venus aspects our natal Venus, even at a hard angle, it often feels soft and sweet. This might be a time when we indulge in adornment and rediscover what makes us feel beautiful, sexy, and beautifully sexy. Tapping into the way we receive pleasure is easier now, and indulging in it as this transit is building is a great idea, as it only lasts a few days.

## Lessons about Self-Love During Venus Retrograde

That old cliché about not being able to love others until you learn to love yourself—it's kind of true, and this lesson is often LOUD during Venus Retrograde phases. Approximately every nineteen months, when Venus descends as an evening star at the start of a Venus Retrograde cycle and then reemerges as a morning star after forty days, we might feel as if we, too, have descended into the deepest reaches of our erotic self-knowledge. (As in Mercury retrograde, Venus doesn't actually move backward in the sky, it just appears to.) Yes, our relationships can go a little pear-shaped during this phase, but only because we're turning inward in ways we usually don't let ourselves, as we often focus on "the other" when we consider what we desire.

I like to think of Venus Retrograde phases as a kind "desire crucible." Plunging to the depths of what we want and renewing this commitment to our desires every nineteen months forces us to redirect our erotic energy and review how we've expended it since the previous Venus Retrograde cycle. It allows us to deepen our erotic self-awareness and put it into practice.

There are myriad ways we can reflect and gain more self-knowledge about our erotic landscape by exploring the beautiful complexity of Venus. This chapter covers signs and some basic transits, but you can also find richness in exploring Venus via house placement, other aspects, and the Venus Start Point. What's the Venus Star Point, you ask? It's a super cool pre-natal point in our charts showing when Venus came together with the Sun in a *cazimi* (an exact conjunction) prior to our birth. This is an area I highly recommend exploring once you've gone more in depth with your Venus. Check out the work of astrologer Arielle Guttman, who wrote the book *The Venus Star Point: Getting Straight to the Heart of Your Life with Venus* for more on this juicy topic.

## An Embodiment Exercise to Receive Venus Energy

This exercise can be used as a companion to the exercise in the Mars chapter or done independently. It can be done anytime, but it may be even more intensely pleasurable and evocative when you or a lover are having a Venus transit. We'll be working with our senses. This can be done naked or clothed.

Come to your sacred space. You can bring honey, lavender petals (or any other flower or fragrant herb, dried or fresh), and some kind of oil, such as olive, coconut, or jojoba.

Light a candle and lie down in a comfortable position with your herbs and oils in reach. Take a few breaths into your second chakra or genital area (see diagram on page 19), visualizing orange light entering your body with the inflow of breath, getting brighter and more defined with every inhale. Imagine this light spilling up your spine with each inhale and down your spine with each exhale, and try to hold the light in your genital area a bit more intensely each time you breathe. Visualize the light hovering there throughout the ritual, warm and glow-y.

Take some flower petals (not all of them) and sprinkle them on the area between your navel and pubic bone, directly on your skin if possible. Every time you work through a different sense, check in with your second chakra and/or your genital area—notice what you feel there.

Begin with sight: close your eyes and try to see an image of your desire. Does it have color or shape? Is it a person you deeply love or an experience? Is it sex you had at some point in your life with someone you may never see again? Is it kissing someone outside of your relationship? Let yourself see whatever is there, and raise your right hand to your third eye for a moment and hold it there (this is the area between your eyebrows).

Now grab some more flower petals. Hold them in your hand and ask yourself: What does my desire smell like? Is there a scent that you can recall, your perfume, someone else's, the smell of a special lover's body, the smell of the ocean or the woods, a spice you cook with? Focus on that smell in your mind, then bring the petals to your nose and inhale their scent.

What does your desire sound like? Is it the voice of a lover, past or present? A sexy love song? The sound of someone's breath or moan? The sound of your own voice while in ecstasy? Hear this sound or make this sound right now.

Take the bottle of oil and pour some into your hand. What does your desire feel like in the tactile sense? As you recall touching something, or someone, or being touched by someone that evoked the heat of your desire, rub some of this oil on your arm or anywhere else that feels right.

What does your desire taste like? Remember something that tasted divinely sexy and turned you on. A favorite food, the salt of someone's skin. Take the honey and let it dissolve on your tongue. Swallow it and see it turning orange as it spills down your spine and chakras and joins the light making your lower belly glow.

Close by taking a few more deep breaths down into your belly, open your eyes if they are closed, and notice how you feel.

# 15

# Mars

## The Pleasure of Pursuit

lust too is a jewel

**Adrienne Rich**

"Two Songs"

**Names of Mars in Other Cultures:** Greek: Ares;
Norse: Tyr; Hindu: Mangala

**Mars Rules:** the fire sign Aries and the
water sign Scorpio

**Color:** Red

**Day of the Week:** Tuesday

**Keywords:** virility, strength, action, forcefulness,
courage, competition, vigor, passion, drive, impulsiveness

Mars, known to the Romans as the god of war, used military force to promote peace. This is quite instructive to those of us learning to work with our own Mars or to negotiate with a lover's Mars. The Roman Mars evolved from the Greek Ares, who was thought of as a more destructive force. Our astrological Mars can both fuck and fight, depending on how he is harnessed.

When the ancients first saw Mars with the naked eye, it glowed blood red, so naturally its assignation was the fierce and feisty warrior god.

We've met Mars in the Aries and Scorpio chapters, as these are the signs he rules—with the hot dagger of cardinal fire in Aries and the deep passionate cauldron of fixed water in Scorpio. In both signs, this warrior planet is meant to always be in pursuit of what it desires, come what may.

I've found that Mars causes more damage when he is not acknowledged, trained, and worked out. He will not sit there idly and wait for us to take him on. Like a bored puppy, Mars will begin ripping up the furniture and barking at the neighbors while we're out enjoying the more socially acceptable parts of our chart.

Natally and by transit, when Mars is healthy (when a person has explored their Mars shadow), he tends to come in hot, moving with initiatory force. As a god, Mars was known for his essential virility and sometimes, savagery. This reputation for savagery is how we get to Mars as a malefic—a planet that can injure us, our beloveds, and our community if we fail to recognize, exercise, and integrate him. Stephen Forrest, in his classic astrology book, *The Inner Sky*, calls Mars' function "assertiveness training." Especially when Mars is a caged and sexually unfed animal, he can be dangerous, destructive, and exhausting. When we feed our Mars a proper erotic diet and take him out for daily walks, he is much better behaved, and his creative, lusty force can take us wherever we want to go.

## The Animal in You

Once again, Mars rules the fire sign Aries and the water sign Scorpio, the two signs most associated with passion, force, and sex. This tells us on one hand that Mars is interested in survival, and to some extent, procreation. Mars rules the genitals and the adrenals—he's in charge of our fight-or-flight mechanism, and this is what can make Mars overreact to stimuli. And if we're going to talk about Mars energy, we must get into the topic of thrusting and phalluses. We're looking at engorgement, erections, blood rushing to areas of the body—I'm speaking of the clitoris and the penis—and swelling with desire. The clitoris is made of the same erectile tissue as the penis, and it grows when we're aroused. In our study of Mars, it's worth exploring the wonders of the clitoris, the only organ in the body that has a singular purpose: pleasure.

Whether alive in the pure physicality of Aries or plunging to Hades in the arms of Scorpio, Mars is not afraid to go down fighting. "Float like a butterfly; sting like a bee," said Muhammad Ali, with his Imum Coeli (the base and one of the most significant angles of the birth chart) deeply rooted in Scorpio.

Pushing, provoking, agitating, inciting: these are a few of the many motivations of Mars energy. The Red Planet is one of the more defiant planets of the astrological pantheon, but I like to think of Mars first in its natural state: as a wild animal enjoying its body. In fact, Mars seems to thrive when movement feels like a game. Like a fencer or a boxer, he does well when he has practiced his skills over and over, exhausting his energy regularly. This is how the lance or the fist can become constructive tools that help us win without causing pain or harm.

## How Mars and Venus Move Together

If Venus receives, as discussed in the previous chapter, Mars lives to deliver. If Venus seduces, Mars actively desires. If Venus softens, Mars hardens. This is how they dance together, energetically, erotically, and sometimes in the ways bodies fit together and interlock. But please note: it is heterosexist garbage to say that men are from Mars and women are from Venus, because all genders have both planets in their charts. You can be a Venus-ruled top or a Mars-ruled bottom or anything in between.

Venus is socially acceptable; Mars is the part of us that polite society often shuns, especially in those socialized as women and labeled "too sexually aggressive" or "slutty." People who live in marginalized bodies with strong or visible Mars energy are often shamed for overt expressions of sexuality. Yet Mars is often used to exploit beauty and desire for advertising dollars. The subversion of Mars using Venusian imagery (this is what "sex sells" does) only pushes the Mars energy available to marginalized bodies further underground, making it more toxic.

Alfred Kinsey, one of the pioneers of the field of sexology and the person who brought us the Kinsey Scale, defined orgasm as "the expulsive discharge of neuromuscular tensions at the peak of the sexual response"— evoking Mars energy in the use of the words "expulsive" and "peak." The moment after orgasm, as we relax in a bath of serotonin, dopamine, and oxytocin, we move back into Venus territory. If our Venus wants to be wanted, it can self-actualize and process its shadow by activating and acting on Mars energy in our chart.

When our Mars is activated, we can find ourselves in a conquering mode. When we are desired, we can feel into our Venus, and when we do the desiring, we are tapping into our Mars, and so forth. Often, in sexual relationships, both of these sensations exist at once, interlinked, forever in a tango. But understanding and exercising each of these astrological "muscles" individually can help us exist in a state of balance between desire, arousal, and release.

Teasing apart the libidinous exchange between Mars and Venus is parsing where desire ends and pleasure begins. Mars (desire, the act of going after) and Venus (pleasure, the experience of receiving what feels good) obviously pair very well together. This is not to say that the experience of raw Mars energy, or raw desire, is bad or dangerous. And certainly, the experience of raw Venus energy, or pleasure not preceded by active desire, is equally as valid, meaningful, and fulfilling.

We can break this down further using the example of spontaneous desire versus responsive desire, concepts first mentioned in the Aries chapter. In Dr. Emily Nagoski's book *Come as You Are*, she explains how responsive desire occurs in response to stimuli, and that it is very common for vulva-havers to experience desire in response to touch. This is in contrast to spontaneous desire, the kind of desire that can be elicited through visual stimuli or through nothing at all. This model is more common for penis-havers, and the model that predominated our understanding of the sexual response cycle for generations. Another way of looking at this is to say that Venus energy is more present (at first) in responsive desire, whereas Mars is more present (at first) in spontaneous desire. These two planetary energies and desire styles then begin to meet in a dance that generates pleasure.

What happens when our Mars instinct is stripped of power or blocked? This might occur when our Mars is under pressure via transit, or we're experiencing something that's affecting our libido. If our natal Mars is weak, we might have to work on this across our lifetime. We might lash out or lay down in surrender, giving up our instinctual fervor in favor of deadening passivity. When Mars is left unexercised and our desires are ignored or abandoned, all that raw energy can turn to aggression and sexual frustration.

What can our Mars placement tell us about how we take our desire for a walk or give it a workout? As mentioned in previous chapters, you can easily find your Mars placement online using astro.com or any number of free astrology apps.

## Mars in Aries

Here, Mars is alive in all his glory, unburdened by doubt. This is the thrusting, jousting, journeying, courageous Mars, sometimes full of just a bit too much wild animal energy for polite societal consumption. This Mars gets his daily walk via active movement and daily (yes, I said DAILY) masturbation or partnered sex. It is a Mars that needs to release in orgasm very regularly, or tensions can mount. Mount is the operative word here—this Mars might like to mount and to be mounted by a lover aggressively (with consent) to feel their inner animal fiercely, yet safely. Dancing is an excellent exercise option for Mars in Aries—even to just one fast-moving house track—and exercise bursts are also great. If this Mars is left to its own devices, it can be prone to sudden eruptions of anger and aggression; this is the shadow they need to work through. Note: this Mars should be careful about being a selfish lover. Make space for partner-pleasing, too.

## Mars in Taurus

When Mars is in a Venus-ruled sign like Taurus, it is compelled, nay propelled, by beauty and sensual gratification. There is no problem here, except that in our modern lives beauty and sensuality aren't always easily accessible. When senses are left unstimulated and the Scorpio shadow (the need for transformation) is ignored, this Mars can grow bored and get stuck in the mud, eventually becoming less able to access their own desire. Mars in Taurus needs fresh flowers in the vase, good smells coming from the kitchen, silky sheets on the bed, self-massage, aromatherapy baths, and various "indulgent" daily activities and exercise to keep it moving—this provides satisfaction and health. Taking those sensorial indulgences and imagining their energy flowing to the genitals can spark erotic bursts of hedonic pleasure that make the Mars in Taurus say, "Yes, please!"

## Mars in Gemini

This Mars has a need for (intellectual) speed. Stimulation of all sorts, from various sources, is what gets Mars in Gemini revved up. In order to move this fast-paced mental energy from the mind to the body, this Mars needs to learn to capture lightning in a bottle, so to speak. This is the realm of intellectual jousting and possibly of mind games, both of which can be turn-ons for Mars in Gemini. However, taking this to the physical realm is the treat that trickster Gemini may find elusive unless they work on their shadow and explore the world around them. Pairing erotic wordplay with touch and stimulation of erogenous zones or directly to the genitals can take this Mars out of the brain and into the body.

## Mars in Cancer

This Mars can have a hard time expressing sexual urges, but that doesn't mean it lacks them! Mars is in its fall in Cancer, a water sign that's generally not comfortable with fiery aggression, so it must work harder to find, acknowledge, and affirm its desires. You know how it's hard to run through waves on the shore? That's what Mars in Cancer can feel like—the inability to know when desire will be huge and daunting one moment, and small and trifling the next. Navigating those peaks and valleys can be emotionally exhausting. The shadow for Mars in Cancer is that security needs can be mixed up with raw animal instinct, and people with this placement may need to work on separating their feelings from the facts of their bodies. At the same time, their Martian superpower is sexual intuition—they often know what their lovers need. Building boundaries in sexual relationships is essential.

## Mars in Leo

Mars in Leo is often able to get to the action fast—so fast that people with this placement can get frustrated with lovers who crave a lot of foreplay or are slower to get down to "Business Time," in Flight of the Conchords parlance. The shadow here is a need for constant affirmation and adoration—a praise fetish that prevents some with this placement from enjoying other sex that doesn't involve intense verbal veneration. Praise play and exhibitionism are great and fun, but Mars in Leo should be on watch to make sure their preferences don't become fixations. Like Mars in Aries, being a selfish lover is possible, just because of the need for instant gratification—otherwise, Leo is a very generous sign. Pacing oneself in solo sessions and shared sexual experiences is necessary.

## Mars in Virgo

One thing that Mars and Virgo have in common is that they both love to have a mission. Yet the shadow here can be a fear of letting go and being completely in the body, because attention must be paid to getting everything perfect. Virgo is an earth sign that is ostensibly grounded in material, sensual touch, but when Mars is here, there can be neurosis and anxiety that decreases sexual pleasure. Once Mars in Virgo sets the scene and makes sure the sheets are unwrinkled, it can pour itself into a raw desire nature and allow itself to get dirty. One secret is that this Mars often loves dirty talk; this is where the kink is in the details.

## Mars in Libra

Mars is in detriment in Libra, as it is the ruler of Aries, its opposite sign. The warrior planet isn't the most comfortable in this more passive place and must work harder to find its erotic mojo. Airy Libra craves beauty and equanimity, fairness, and justice, and when Mars is here, desire for *ideas* can sometimes supersede desire for sexual pleasure and consummation. This is where the Mars in Libra shadow can get caught up. People with this placement can be immensely charming, so much so that it entrances would-be lovers. However, without actively exploring their animal instincts, people with this placement may fear passion, faking desire instead of feeling it.

## Mars in Scorpio

The word "intense" is wholly overused in regard to all things Scorpio (I am guilty of this, even in this book!), but with this placement the descriptor applies with almost surgical precision. Mars in Scorpio smolders with desire, and it can be a bit intimidating to potential lovers. In the act of shared sex or solo sex, a transformation can take place, seemingly transmuting those involved into a different form of matter. When Mars is in Scorpio, orgasm can feel like entering a space-time portal and landing in a different dimension, forever changed by overwhelming, intense consumption and pleasure. Were this to happen every day, it might be exhausting, so people with this placement may do better pacing themselves. The shadow here is control: attempting to "have" a particular lover or obsessively and insistently pushing sexual desire or fantasy on an existing lover.

## Mars in Sagittarius

For Mars in Sagittarius, sex can be positive, affirmative, and wildly hilarious. Here, the final fire sign, ruled by Jupiter, gets to go big and dive into eroticism with gusto. This can make for very athletic, fun sex, but not necessarily deeply intimate, emotionally connected sex. This is not to say that those with this placement aren't capable of that level of intimacy, of course—just that when their Mars is activated, they may be more interested in being thrown around (or doing the throwing) than staring into a lover's eyes and feeling their heartbeat. Mars in Sagittarius can wear their partners out. Their shadow is boredom—they may feel like they need a sexual relationship to expand exponentially and evolve on its own, and when it doesn't, their desire can lag.

## Mars in Capricorn

Power meets power when Mars comes to Capricorn. The forcefulness of the warrior planet can feel more sustainable in this practical sign, where Mars is exalted. This Mars placement feels an ease about the way its body moves through the world and can find a sense of grounding and sensuality in situations where people with different placements might feel a bit out of control. When this sign gives even a small bit of their time to their erotic life, it can be tremendously fulfilling and satisfying. The shadow here is being so overly ambitious about worldly success that they forget how important it is to tend to their body and a lover's body. They should schedule in sex, solo or partnered, so they don't forget, but when they do make time for it, they must avoid being overly goal-oriented.

## Mars in Aquarius

Mars is in fixed air when it is in Aquarius, and before it can reach for sexual satisfaction, it must first feel truly free. This is probably one of the most liberated and liberating Mars placements and exudes a kind of cool, calm, and collected uniqueness when it comes to erotic pursuits. Highly intellectual and curious, Mars in Aquarius is often attracted to those who are brilliant and different—lovers they can get weird and be themselves with. For solo sex, they can experience extreme pleasure using sex tech and tend to be very comfortable exploring the latest gadgetry. The shadow of this placement is emotional detachment to the extreme. They are capable of cutting off their feelings even in situations that feel deeply intimate to their partners, and this can be disconcerting and confusing. Leaning into logic can help Mars in Aquarius unpack their erotic longings better than focusing first on feelings.

## Mars in Pisces

This is one of those Mars placements that needs to be regularly reminded that it has sexual organs, as it can reach for eroticism that is more ethereal than real and embodied. Mars in the sign of the Fishes gives off sexy vibes and feels spiritual connections to other humans that it may interpret as sexual attraction. The shadow here can be a fear of assertiveness that prevents sexual connection and communion altogether—they may be intimidated about approaching others, thinking it's too coarse and vulgar to express sexual desire or interest. Mars in Pisces tends to be delicate in sensibility, so exploring their desires first in fantasy, then bringing the body along may be the best course of action. This can help them to wake up their erotic energy, so they can use it regularly in real life.

## Managing Transits to the Natal Mars

As discussed in the previous chapter, transits happen when planets in orbit make mathematical angles to our natal placements, activating certain themes in our lives. Being aware of transits to our Mars can help to harness our aggression, alert us to peak or low libido phases, and let us know when and how we might try to transmute our anger into a healthier kind of passion. As in the Venus chapter, I'm only including the harder aspects here, and using transits from the outer/transpersonal planets, plus Venus and Mars.

## Pluto

When transiting Pluto makes a conjunction, square, or opposition to our natal Mars, it can feel like a nuclear explosion is gradually erupting from deep within our bodies. This is a slow transit during which our instinctual selves may rumble like a volcano taking years to spew lava, allowing new forms to take shape deep below the boiling fire. This can allow us to grapple with some of our more unseemly sexual impulses and expunge powerful layers of shame.

## Neptune

When Neptune contacts our natal Mars, it can deplete, confuse, and exhaust our erotic energy reserves as we search for spiritual meaning in our sexual relationships. It can completely melt away boundaries around our sovereign sexual self and make us feel a bit invisible in our intimate partnerships. If we do enter fantasy worlds under this transit, we might feel frustration and even rage when we realize we can't get what we want in the real world.

## Uranus

A craving for instant change can shake up even the most grounded sense of our sexual self. This might feel like a come-from-nowhere, is-this-really-me type of sensation. It can spark sudden, unexpected anger, attractions and affairs, or out-of-the-blue breakups because one partner or the other no longer feels passion—or has found that passion elsewhere, instantaneously. Finding sources of sexual stimulation that don't wholly rock our boats and throw us over the edge is helpful when Uranus comes at our natal Mars. We feel like we must rebel, but doing it safely, while calming the nervous system, is essential.

## Saturn

When Saturn meets with our natal Mars, it might feel like restriction, or a force that requires us to impose restraint on our sexual impulses. There can be a deadening of our desires now, but if we tune into the absence of ardor, we might find that we need to make a change, perhaps to our daily habits or our relationships, in order to bring back lagging passions. This can help us to get serious about our sexual issues and do what it takes to bring back any vitality that has been lost.

## Jupiter

A surge of optimism and excitement can pump up our erotic energy when Jupiter visits with our natal Mars. Even the more challenging aspects—the square and opposition—can feel pretty damn good. This is like a shot in the arm for passion, and it can feel particularly positive if it comes after a difficult period. We may, to put it mildly, be very horny during this time, and whether we're single or involved, we may need to find ways to scratch that itch, over and over, and over again.

## Mars

When transiting Mars hits our natal Mars, it can impact us like fireworks or friction, depending on the way our sex lives are feeling at the moment. Anger and frustration can be high, yet tuning into our raw physical needs can alleviate the irritation rather easily. This might mean exercising more, but it might also mean engaging our base instincts and having what some might call "animalistic" sex with a willing partner, or just fantasizing about it with release. We should watch out for bursts of anger and avoid frustrating people and situations.

## Venus

When Venus awakens Mars, our sensual selves can roar with desire. As his cosmic consort beckons, even with a hard aspect, it can feel like an urgency from the part of us that knows what it wants and is willing to do whatever it takes to get it. No matter what our relationship status, our sex lives are usually on our minds at this time, and we might be more interested in adornment and the accoutrements of dating and romance to stir up passion within or without.

## An Embodiment Exercise to Awaken Mars Energy

This ritual can be done in conjunction with the Venus ritual in the previous chapter or independently. If done together, it works well to start with the Venus ritual and finish with the Mars ritual. This ritual can be performed naked or clothed. It calls for an oil, and any will do, but if you have a warming sensual oil, one made for arousal, that might hit the spot.

Come to or remain in your sacred space. If you performed the Venus ritual first, remove the flower petals from your belly if they're still there. Lying down or sitting comfortably, bring your awareness to your second chakra and your genital area—your vulva, clitoris, penis, anus, perineum, your lower belly, or your inner thighs. If you've become acquainted with your personal erogenous zones by reading this book, consider bringing your attention to them as well.

Take a few audible, assertive breaths down into your genitals and visualize pulling those breaths up through your crown chakra as you exhale. These can be quickened breaths, but do try to remain relaxed. Simply feel into your genital region for a few minutes, letting your awareness hover there. Does it feel vitalized, alive, tingly, active, *ready*? Take some of the oil in your hand and rub it on your lower belly, massaging around your navel just to the edge of your genitals.

How do you feel? If you feel connected to your desire now, can you note where and how you felt aroused first, and how it peaked into more active desire? Or did you begin feeling desire before you touched yourself? Are you still waiting for desire to happen? If so, you can start from the beginning of the Venus ritual, tuning into any of your senses that felt like they needed more attention.

This dual ritual is a wonderful prelude to partnered or solo sex—and it can bring a different, more intense, more alive, vital orgasm. If you choose this experience and have an orgasm, note whether it is different than ones you've had in the past. If possible, without overthinking, try to tune into your senses through the entire experience.

# 16

# Black Moon Lilith

### The Pleasure of Rejecting Shame and Reclaiming Sexual Power

I will not lie below.

**Lilith to Adam**

*Alphabet of Ben Sira*

F*ck the pain away

**Peaches**

*The Teaches of Peaches*

Black Moon Lilith is not a planet like Mars or Venus. Rather, it's the apogee or furthest point of the Moon's orbit from the Earth in a natal chart—essentially, it's a dark void in space. Some astrologers, like me, believe this point tells us a lot about our secret, subversive, and hidden desires. Black Moon Lilith is energetically connected to the Earth's center, and it symbolizes the darkest hidden depths that we must dig deep into in order to root out and explore. It is completely shrouded by darkness and "blacked out"—opposite to what we are accustomed to making conscious. In this way, Black Moon Lilith serves as a kind of foil for the Sun—offering a deeper investigation into the most intense and provocative of our sexual shadows.

Lilith, in our charts, shows us precisely what we may have repressed because our white supremacist heteropatriarchy tells us it's disallowed. You can find your courage, ferocity, and sexual confidence in this place by doing some work to unearth it.

To be frank, I LOVE LILITH. I would say without exaggeration that Lilith is one of my top three favorite astrological placements, so forgive me if I wax poetic and effusive in this chapter. She's my home girl, my bestie, my ride-or-die. From my astrological perspective, Lilith's main promise and purpose is to give marginalized bodies access to their desires, and that is why I adore her.

## Where's Your Black Moon Lilith?

I'll be using the shorthand "Lilith" here for a more specific point in our charts—Black Moon Lilith. This can get confusing, because three separate objects or astronomical points, all called Lilith, are recognized in astronomy and astrology. This complex, mysterious backstory really goes with Lilith's subversive nature! There is Lilith the asteroid, Dark Moon Lilith (a potential second Moon that circles Earth, one that has never been proven to exist), and Black Moon Lilith, the astronomical point I'm writing about here. Most astrologers mean Black Moon Lilith when they talk about Lilith these days. You can find yours in most astrology software, or for free at astro.com by going to the extended chart selection and choosing Lilith under "additional objects."

## Lilith's Mythological History

When I explain the import of a natal Lilith placement to a client in a reading, I begin with the Jewish Lilith, drawn in part from folklore and mythology, telling the story of her journey as Adam's first wife. If you think Eve's apple-eating behavior was subversive and she was inappropriately punished, you're not going to believe what happened to Lilith. In the *Alphabet of Ben Sira*, a rabbinic text from the Middle Ages, it says that Lilith was *equal* to Adam—made from the same clay.[1]

Jewish folklore suggests that Lilith was banished from the garden. In my imagination, Adam wanted Lilith to obey him, and because she was horny and had desires, she said, "Fuck that noise," and left the garden to live on the beaches with the demons, so she could conduct her sex life exactly as she pleased.

The folklore says that Adam asked God to replace Lilith, and because he didn't want to risk making the "from the same clay" mistake again, he made Eve from Adam's rib, so she would be forced to obey him and to lay beneath him.

Eve, on the other hand, was brainwashed (in my opinion) into believing she came from a rib. Still: she reached for the apple. She reached for it, and she took a bite, because she was hungry, perhaps for knowledge, perhaps for the fruit itself. Maybe she listened to her body in that moment, not to Adam and not to God. According to biblical scholars, her punishment was centuries of shame and physical pain, of women choking back their desires, being afraid to even ask themselves about their sexual nature, and of accepting far less than their fair share of pleasure. But Lilith, both in our myths and in our charts, symbolizes our righteous rage about all of that.

What if Lilith's leave-taking was a form of *self-banishment* as a rejection of patriarchal values? I believe Lilith, not derived from Adam's rib, fully had a mind of her own, so she refused to obey. If Lilith was angry because Adam wanted her to be subservient, and she wanted to be on top—both literally and metaphorically, well, I'm angry too. She demanded that her desires be recognized, and that's why I love her so damn much. In another telling of her myth, she is known as the mother of Adam's demonic progeny after he separated from Eve—these children are known as *incubi* and *succubi*.

In Hebrew, Lilith can translate to "night monster," and the writers of the Torah/Bible and some of their Midrashic interpreters (that is to say, the writers of the early history of patriarchy) certainly made Lilith into a monster, simply because she demanded bodily autonomy and pleasure. In the Zohar Leviticus, she was called "a hot fiery female who first cohabitated with man."[2] Needless to say, that sounds close to the way right-wing politicians describe those of us who believe in equal rights for marginalized bodies, like the right to abortion, birth control, and sex education.

Before the Hebrew Bible was written, Lilith appeared in Sumerian mythology as the handmaid of the goddess Inanna, the Queen of Heaven. Lilith assists Inanna when she has to go deep underground to save her sister. Lilith's presence in the Bible was, in fact, likely derived from a class of Mesopotamian demons. Although scholars aren't exactly sure when the myth of Lilith emerged and from where, many believe she was inspired by Sumerian myths about female vampires. This is possibly why one of my favorite classic HBO series, *True Blood*, made Lilith into the mother of all vampires. In other words, whatever her exact origins, Lilith is extremely powerful, extremely disorienting to the regular order of society, and extremely intriguing precisely because she is so subversive.

In the way that early pagan gods, goddesses, and rituals were often subsumed by monotheistic religions, eventually, Lilith became Christianity's dangerous sex demon and is often talked about that way even today. Her refusal to be submissive cast her lot in the patriarchal power plays of the Bible and most of the Western culture that grew out of it.

This, to me, shows how threatened patriarchal forces have always been by those who dare to demand their bodily autonomy. In *Ulysses*, James Joyce called Lilith "the patron of abortions," further evidence of why we all need Lilith energy in our lives now, as our bodily freedoms remain in peril. I would add that Lilith seems to be the patron of sex workers, drag queens, and anyone who works with subversive versions of sexuality and gender.

The myth of Lilith has been reclaimed by feminists for the last five decades or so, perhaps first and most notably in a 1972 piece in *Ms.* by Lilly Rivlin called, simply, "LILITH." There is also the fantastic Jewish feminist literary magazine, *Lilith*, calling us back to her astonishing reclamation of power.

The feminist reclamation speaks to the centuries during which women were burned as witches, corseted, enslaved by marriage, and called "hysterical" for daring to express any sexual desire. This is the rebellion of the Lilith archetype, shaking it all up. Because Lilith is in the charts of all genders, she represents the same rebellious, primal archetype for all people.

Lilith is often associated with our inner "bitch," regardless of our gender, but if we're going to use that phrase, we're going to have to seriously reappropriate it. She is a bitch perhaps, but a righteous bitch. Her rage is understandable—she's been cut off and cast out simply because she dared to be in her body, to own her needs, and to refuse to submit. Once we know where Lilith lives in our own chart, we may start to refuse to submit to anyone who would dampen our instinctual power in that precise way.

## Black Moon Lilith as the Source of Our Secret, Hidden Sexual Power

Another way to get inside our Lilith is to imagine its position in our charts as the source of our unconscious desires, hidden drives, and buried elements of our psyche. I like to think of our Black Moon Lilith as our *unbridled, raw sexuality, and creativity*. However, (and this is important) if we don't actively integrate our Lilith into our lives and make her conscious, she might harm us by making us feel rageful and self-sabotaging.

When Black Moon Lilith energy is suppressed, it can send us into an intense and uncontrollable rage. It requires the oxygen of consciousness raising, that seventies second-wave feminist tool (reimagined for the age of intersectional feminism), to awaken as a force for reclamation. Many people spend their whole lives without ever meeting, interrogating, and integrating their Black Moon Lilith. Those people may miss out on their deepest desires.

## Stop Repressing Your Black Moon Lilith: Lilith in Your Chart

Our Black Moon Lilith can be suppressed and ignored because we feel ashamed of it. We learn quickly, as children, but especially by puberty and adolescence, that our Black Moon Lilith instincts can be dangerous and not suitable for public consumption. Yet we can use our unique Black Moon Lilith placement to upend all of that, peeling back shame and blame.

When your Lilith is named, recognized, understood, and expressed, her energy can feel like healthy passion and deep empowerment depending on what sign she is in. When she is repressed and denied, she will express rage, resentment, and fury, as typified by her sign in your chart. She shows you where your fears are your strength, and where your hidden desires reveal an ultimate truth about your sexual power. Tapping into our Black Moon Lilith placement can help us integrate our inner rebel, setting us on a shame-free path to reclaimed sexuality.

Depending on where Lilith was at the time of your birth, she will express herself differently, and have different strengths, weaknesses, and desires. You can delve deeper if you look at the house placement and aspects Lilith makes to other planets. But knowing her basic approach, which is to say her sign placement, gives us a lot to work with as we begin to integrate her into our daily lives.

## Lilith in Aries

Lilith in Aries is pure ferocity—this might feel like fear of anger soothed by the power of authentic love. She rebels against anyone or anything she feels is trying to stop her from expressing herself fully. She may come across as impolite or rude, too physically imposing or demanding, too raw. You may have anger issues, or have had early life experiences that featured repressed anger or domestic violence if you were born in this position. It can be difficult to express strength, but this can be liberated by embracing healthy, truly equal sexual relationships.

## Lilith in Taurus

You can become sensuality and decadence incarnate with Lilith in Taurus, or, alternatively, live in fear of lack. Before this Lilith is liberated, it might feel like nothing is enough, including sensorial experiences and pleasure. This Lilith may feel ashamed about having too much or too little. She is completely free once she understands that she has an innate and instinctual sense of self-worth that cannot be bought or manipulated, and owns her bodily autonomy hungrily and proudly.

## Lilith in Gemini

When Lilith is in Gemini, you may fear being silenced, but also may secretly resent not being allowed to express your innate genius. Or, you may be plagued by doubt and shame about your intelligence. Speaking your sexual truth out loud and talking about desire publicly may be the key to this Lilith's liberation. Owning the power of this Lilith placement may require demanding a platform that will allow your higher truth to shine through. You can say whatever you want, whenever you like, once you are brave enough to shout your truth from the rooftops—especially when it's the truth about your desire.

## Lilith in Cancer

If you were born while Lilith was in Cancer, your deepest shame might be a fear of abandonment, but it can be liberated by the power of self-nurturing. You may tend to cling to the nearest human for dear life, afraid of being left alone. It's not uncommon to desperately want someone to give you some old-fashioned maternal love. Your sexual liberation comes when you allow yourself to love without fear of being left and without guilt about being "too much" for anyone.

## Lilith in Leo

This Lilith may long to be in the spotlight, but carries deep shame about this desire and waits backstage, feeling more and more rage. This might be a secret fantasy about exhibitionism that is buried deep in the psyche. This Lilith placement can instead live in a state of perceived invisibility or obscurity. Falling in love with yourself authentically, knowing in your heart of hearts that you are worthy of adoration and applause—that's where the liberation lives. Once you're willing to flaunt your sexual skills or work as an artist or another kind of public figure, you can find and embrace that radical self-love that sets you free.

### Lilith in Virgo

Lilith in Virgo may live with a deep-seated fear of chaos, losing control of sexual sovereignty and their own body, causing hypervigilance around desire that can turn to rage. Not having enough concrete information about sexuality can cause resentment, but your mind is the key to liberation—once you realize that the only moment you're in control of is the current one, and the only body you're in control of is your own, you are set free. Also helpful: finding books, documentaries, courses, and other informational sources about sexuality—in other words, becoming an expert.

### Lilith in Libra

Lilith in Libra can create a powerful fear of being alone, one that is liberated by authentic independence. There can be dependence on romantic partnerships that eventually causes toxicity, resentment, and sexual shutdown. Family, culture, and early childhood messaging may have pushed the idea that having an "other half" is your only salvation. This Lilith may need to do just as the mythological Lilith did—live independently for a time, having a wide range of sexual experiences outside of the bounds of commitment.

### Lilith in Scorpio

This Lilith placement often fears emotional vulnerability so much that they stop expressing desire, just so that they can't be rejected. The depths of power are so consuming here that they may scare people into a kind of flat, desireless space of playing small and not asking for much. Learning how to express desires without shame is what this Lilith needs for liberation. Just saying the words "I want" can be challenging but deeply rewarding.

### Lilith in Sagittarius

This Lilith was born deeply curious, but something (culture, parents, religion) may have nipped that curiosity in the bud, directing them to stop asking so many questions. Stripped of intellectual agency and the ability to explore and experience sexual adventure, this Lilith needs to dig deep to liberate themselves from the clutches of patriarchal customs and mores. Rebelling for rebellion's sake might be tempting, but true freedom exists in deep interrogation of one's own stultifying roots.

## Lilith in Capricorn

Those born with Lilith in Capricorn can become control freaks as adults, especially if they didn't receive proper nurturing from guardians as a child. They may feel wholly sexually responsible for their partners, but secretly long to have someone else take over so they can rest. Their liberation lies in knowing they don't have to do everything all the time to maintain an emotional or sexual bond—they are allowed to relax.

## Lilith in Aquarius

Lilith in Aquarius can be a total nonconformist in the sexual realm, yet retain the idea that it's dangerous to be different, keeping themselves flat, inert, and invisible. Exploring and exploding myths about kink and queerness is essential to liberate this Lilith, even if it turns out their desires are rather vanilla. Finding and embracing their inner rebel and isolating their uniqueness can eventually become their superpower, as can finding their chosen family.

## Lilith in Pisces

Lilith in Pisces might find their sexual liberation in exploring their dreams and psychic abilities, something they may have been taught to ignore or repress. There can be a sexual voraciousness that remains fully in the realm of fantasy here, and in order to experience a deeper self-knowledge and satisfaction, they may need to create active, directed engagement with these inner realms and draw out those fantasies using dream journaling, meditation, and/or learn to harness lucid dreaming techniques.

## An Embodiment Exercise to Engage with Your Lilith

### Active Imagination Ritual

Come to your altar or other sacred space with a notebook. Sit down and take five slow, deep breaths into your belly or genital region. Say one or all of the following statements. See if your Lilith agrees, answers, or tells you which one you might need to expand upon. Write down the dialogue.

"I have an opinion, and I will express it without reservation."

"I have sexual needs, and I will satisfy them."

"I am in this room, and you will look at me, because I am not ashamed to take up space."

"My body is mine, and it's damn f*cking sexy."

"I am NOT sorry."

"GET OUT OF MY WAY."

# Conclusion

## The Liberation in Your Stars

Another world is not only possible, she is on her way. Maybe
many of us won't be here to greet her, but on a quiet day,
if I listen very carefully, I can hear her breathing.

**Arundhati Roy**

"Come September"

The continuously evolving fields of sexuality and astrology, both
taboo subjects at various moments in history, are experiencing a
colossal renaissance. It's beyond thrilling for me to live and work at the
intersection of these two disciplines.

Never has there been a moment when humans had so much direct
access to shame-smashing knowledge about their bodies, their desires,
and the way the planets may influence them. We are several decades
into a golden age of information about both sex and astrology, but at
the same time, conservative crackdowns and backlash are growing more
intense in response to the kinds of liberation we seek.

Radical right-wing culture wars have led to dangerous anti-
LGBTQIA+ legislation, book bans, a renewed assault on reproductive
rights, attempts to dismantle democracy, and all the other horrors we've
faced late in the first quarter of the twenty-first century. Marginalized
groups and their allies have fought these fascist forces for what seems like
forever, and the struggle continues.

No matter how the political pendulum shifts back and forth, these
cruel ideologies never seem to truly go away, and they won't until we
*wholly* dismantle the complex systemic sources of oppression that have

been coming after people for centuries. There's a lot of work to be done to protect our vulnerable communities, but I see hope for change in the astrology of the decades ahead.

Whether I'm studying personal transits or world events, as an astrologer, the question I'm always asking myself is "Why now?" Generally, astrologers look at the transpersonal or outer planets to gauge historical events. This branch of astrology is called "Mundane" or "World Astrology." There is a wonderful book by Richard Tarnas called *Cosmos and Psyche: Intimations of a New World View* that I highly recommend to anyone who wants to better understand how planetary cycles have intersected with history.

The first-ever American Pluto Return[1] brought an unimaginable rending of the American consciousness as we lived through a global pandemic, a much-needed racial reckoning, and barely survived the collapse of democracy. Pluto eviscerates whatever it touches, transforming it into a new kind of matter. I liken Pluto transits to our natal planets being slowly run over by a tank, and after being flattened over several years, having to rebuild ourselves out of dust, creating a whole new cellular structure. But Pluto is so slow-moving that human beings never experience a Pluto return like the United States, a global superpower, did about 250 years after it was born. So what remnants are in the dust of the past from which our collective can rebuild itself in the next few decades?

The generation-altering planetary event of right now and our future is Pluto's transit through Aquarius through the 2040s. We're looking at an era that will be defined by technology—our relationship to robots and bots, artificial intelligence, and all things not of human origin. The last transit of Pluto through the sign of Aquarius brought us the beginning of the Industrial Revolution and its intersection with an era of rebellion—the Age of Revolutions. I suspect that global uprisings may also be a dominant theme, but hopefully with love at the center of it all.

Even as technology advances and touches more of our lives and bodies, we will need to cleave to the knowledge that we are mammals over and over and over again. Think about how many of us already wake up and reach immediately for our phones instead of reacclimating to our own body in the bed, before sighing or stretching, before taking in the sounds around us, or touching a lover or pet sleeping next to us. As technology reaches deeper into our bodies to the point where we go from wearing it to implanting it, it may further divorce us from our instinctual relationship to desire and pleasure—our mammalian, animal self.

The natural world has given us the astrology we know. As the climate emergency worsens and the environment our bodies understand disappears, we must remember it. As we're forced to spend more time inside during pandemics, wildfires, and floods, the loneliness epidemic we are already experiencing may get worse.

Pluto in Aquarius may give us technology to replace what our animal bodies desire, but let's keep in mind that Leo, the opposite sign of Aquarius, is the shadow of this era: our hearts must come along for the ride too. During Pluto's last transit through Aquarius, the incessant progress of technology spawned microcultures of rebellion, including Romanticism. I wouldn't be shocked if we fall in love with poetry all over again in the coming years. Who will be our new Percy Bysshe Shelley? Community care, the clarion call of the Pluto in Aquarius age, is something we'll need to continue to organize and fight for in the years ahead.

The dangers of disinformation and conspiracy theories online show us how our golden age of Aquarian information might be fraught with peril, even as it offers us deep, nourishing wisdom and practical advice from trained experts. It's up to us to navigate these spaces with careful, skeptical judgment and to make sure our sources are qualified—including in the realms of sex and astrology.

## The Future of Astrology

The cultural resurgence of astrology is nearly impossible to avoid, so much so that I expect there may be a backlash in the coming years. This has happened many times in history—astrology had been a dominant cultural force during various eras and then vanished, only to emerge again. Under the Pluto in Aquarius transit that will take us through the next few decades, science and technology will be at the forefront of our lives, and practices and paradigms that have not been rigorously sub-jected to the scientific method may be shunned.

Astrology certainly doesn't require this kind of vetting to be taken seriously, because it's not making a scientific claim or commentary. Yet it's possible, of course, for the astrology community to begin collecting, collating, and measuring our data to show proof of concept. Personally, I'd be happy to see us put it to the test.

Astrology is now so ubiquitous that during the last dozen years or so, at parties, over dinners, on park benches, people have been talking about their planetary placements and transits, and those of their friends, family, colleagues, partners, and would-be lovers. It's long been said that "the internet is made of cats," but I'd offer that it is now made of both cats and astrology content.

As a long-time professional counseling astrologer, I'm deeply heart-ened to see the field I've studied and fought to defend since the late nineties finally getting its due in the United States (in places like India, astrology has long been a part of daily life). This is tremendously empow-ering for people experiencing patterns they can't seem to shake, even with years of therapy.

Simply put, astrology helps us see the energetic shape of both our pain and our potential. In this way, it shows us how to heal the past and forge a path forward. It's an invaluable supplementary resource to all the other tools we might use for sexual healing, including sex coaching, sex therapy, couples counseling, and mind-body modalities like meditation, yoga, and tantra teachings. Whether it's used for psychological analy-sis, spiritual insight, or relationship repair, astrology offers a potent tool for experiential self-knowledge and discovery, even for those who once resisted it for fear of being too "out there."

Yet I still hear from clients, subscribers to my Substack column, and people who slip into my DMs, that they want to talk to their long-time astrologers about sex and the body—but it's not always comfortable. There is nothing more central to creating and maintaining a healthy, safe, fulfilling sex life than communication. Seeing communication in action is one of the reasons people adore Esther Perel, author of *Mating in*

*Captivity*, and Orna Guralnik, the therapist at the center of the smash hit *Couples Therapy*—they both speak plainly and compassionately about the fundamental necessity of talking about sex, every day, in every way.

There is another layer of complexity here. If an astrologer, psychotherapist, or other clinician hasn't done self-investigative work around their own sexuality, they may not be very comfortable talking about *your* sexuality, as they may still be dealing with their own shame. This is not to say that your current, amazing counselor or anyone you've worked with in the past sucks at their job—it's just to say that sexuality remains a third rail that most professions aren't fully equipped to confront. Cultural, religious, and other kinds of shame have done a number on all of us—even the wisest, most intuitive healers we know.

Similar to the way some therapists react to their clients' concerns about sexuality, or the way many gynecologists won't discuss waning libidos or sexual concerns that come up during perimenopause, counseling astrologers often silo sexuality off for someone else to deal with. They might point to a hard aspect between Venus and Pluto or a fifth house issue and shy away from interrogating a possible sexual concern, simply because of their own discomfort or because they don't feel like they have the language to deal with it. Or worse, they might further shame a client already worrying about whether their sexual functioning is normal. Not intentionally, of course—but just because they aren't sure how to talk about it.

I know from discussions with astrology colleagues that they often feel uneasy talking about sexuality with clients, because we haven't yet carved out a professional space for this to happen with adequate boundaries and safety. In my clinical sexology and sex coaching program, one of the most important projects I did was conducting my own sexual self-assessment. It was powerful, intense, insightful, and very challenging. I highly encourage my colleagues and students of astrology to do this, and to consider doing a few sessions with a sex coach or clinical sexologist.

Generally, I find that my younger Millennial and Gen Z clients are more comfortable asking direct questions about sex, unless they come from a very religious or conservative background. Younger astrologers, too, seem more broadly equipped to have these conversations, which is a relief, but the landscape around this topic remains problematic.

## Astrology and Shame

How do we give astrology the staying power so many of us feel that it deserves, so that we can avoid the backlash I mentioned earlier? In part, by addressing the inherent shame that some still feel while seeking its counsel or practicing it. I'm happy to see that this continues to shift, but even more can be done to normalize it so it doesn't become an out-of-date trend in the coming years.

Once upon a time, successful, smart, and overeducated New York City professionals came into my home office and told me that our astrology session was a secret that they'd guard for life. This was often the case for women with cis-male partners—they didn't want husbands or boyfriends to know they'd consulted with an astrologer. In addition, during the first fifteen years of my career, my consultations were with about ninety-five percent women. During the last five years or so, many cishet men have begun to come in seeking astrology counseling. This is a paradigm shift!

These days, clients often come to me knowing their chart basics. This is usually a bonus, yet sometimes I must undo a bit of "fake news" about their chart, usually something they learned online or from a friend. This is one drawback to the explosion of astrology in our culture: there are a lot of scammers feeding dangerous misinformation into the knowledge ecosystem. From YouTube to TikTok to Instagram and Twitter/X, not to mention Facebook, there are charlatans out there trying to make a buck without the time, focus, and intense study it takes to practice astrology.

It takes many years to become a competent astrologer, yet some people think reading a few articles and watching a few YouTube tutorials is enough. When you're dealing with something as delicate as a person's psyche and working with their trauma and relationship history, you need counseling experience: you can't just watch TikTok videos and "figure it out." Always vet your astrologer, and don't be afraid to ask questions about where, how, and when they learned what they claim to know.

## Transform Now or Get Left Behind

For me, reinforcing that pleasure is sacred—as important as breathing—is one way to both remember that I am a human animal and also ensure that I'm in touch with my heart. It's easy to forget the primacy of your body even when you're just holding a smartphone in your hand. There is a lot to unpack here, especially when we consider the myriad ways technology already touches and will continue to touch our lives.

It remains to be seen if our world will be reborn again in justice, fairness, and pleasure for all during the Pluto in Aquarius era. To me, part of pleasure activism is creating spaces in which we all feel safe, and navigating through Pluto in Aquarius will likely amp up our need to build these spaces together.

Why end a book about sexual astrology with a postscript about the astrology of these difficult, fraught times? Because there has never been a better time for knowing the whole self so that we can be a part of a collective reimagining. You cannot have economic, racial, and gender justice without sexual liberation, and you cannot have collective liberation unless we all look at our individual shadows.

Astrology, if it teaches us anything, shows how to work with our shadows and use them to transform our lives and heal our trauma. Together, we can rebuild the world and experience plenty of pleasure while we're at it.

# Sexual Pleasure Self-Assessment

When we start working together, I ask my clients to complete a Sexual Pleasure intake form to help us better understand where they've come from, where they are now, and what they hope for in the future. I'm sharing this Sexual Pleasure Self-Assessment tool here in case it's helpful for you in working with *Sex and Your Stars*. I encourage you to explore these questions in a journal or another safe space. If you're not comfortable writing, you can try speaking your answers into a voice recorder or just reflecting to yourself. Take your time—no need to answer these questions quickly—and there are no right or wrong answers, just your answers!

What does the word *pleasure* mean to me?

Do I experience *some kind of pleasure* every day—not necessarily from solo or partnered sex?

What is my relationship to my body, right now, in this moment?

Am I sensually attuned to my environment?

Am I having the kind of sex I want to be having, either with myself or with a lover?

Have I experienced any sexual trauma or other kinds of trauma that has impacted my relationship to my body?

What is my first memory of sexual pleasure?

What was my first partnered sexual experience?

Did shame follow my first memory of sexual pleasure or my first partnered sexual experience?

How much stress am I experiencing on a daily basis?

How is that stress affecting my libido? How is that stress affecting the sex I'm having with myself or a partner?

Has my interest in sex waxed or waned in the last six months? Twelve months? Two years?

When I think about sexual experiences from earlier in my life, am I longing to reclaim pleasure that feels "lost"? Or am I longing to have even better sex than I did then?

In addition to the inital sexual self-assessment, at some point in our work together, I ask clients to take a hand mirror and look at their genitals, then write a bit about what they see and feel. Consider adding that step to this self-assessment.

# Acknowledgments

I am deeply grateful to Dr. Patti Britton, the mother of sex coaching, for her mentorship, friendship, and the extensive wisdom she has shared with me about the wide world of sexology. My time at Sex Coach U during the pandemic is the blessing that gave birth to this book.

I am forever indebted to my long-time agent and friend Jennifer Unter, who has helped me shepherd my wild ideas into books for more than twenty years. I'm immensely grateful to my talented and kind editor Sarah Stanton for her insight, and for helping shape my vision for *Sex in Your Stars* into a book that I'm proud of.

I'm beyond thankful to all my astrology colleagues and teachers from whom I continue to learn every day, and will for the rest of my life. A *very special*, huge thanks to my dear friend, the brilliant astrologer Stephanie Gailing, for her wisdom about these pages! I thank my lovers (you know who you are) for teaching me what it means to live in a body and to share it, and for helping me to unravel erotic mysteries over the course of my life.

Most of all, I want to thank my clients for their honesty, bravery, strength, and resilience, and for their willingness to go on a journey to sexual self-knowledge and pleasure with me. You are my teachers, too.

# Notes

## Introduction

1  During the European Renaissance, astrologers and astronomers were often one and the same. Galileo Galilei is probably the most famous of them.

2  Before that, in the nineties, profound scholarship about ancient astrology was undertaken by Robert Hand (one of the preeminent astrologers of our time) and his colleagues. Project Hindsight uncovered and translated ancient texts that gave twenty-first-century astrologers access to the very roots of Western or tropical astrology—and the foundation of Hellenistic astrology was accessible to all.

3  This insight becomes even more valuable if we consider what traditional astrology calls the *sect leader* of our chart—when we know whether the Sun or the Moon is our sect leader, we know which body has a more powerful influence in our lives. You can determine this by noting whether the Sun is in the top or lower half of your natal chart—or by consulting an astrologer or astrology app, because it can become a little tricky when the Sun is near your ascendant.

## Chapter 1: Charting the Sex in Your Stars

1  "Violence Against Women," World Health Organization, last modified March 9, 2021, who.int/news-room/fact-sheets/detail/violence-against-women.

## Chapter 11: Capricorn Sexuality

1  Sharon Olds, *The Dead and the Living* (New York: Alfred A. Knopf, 1990).

## Chapter 16: Black Moon Lilith

1   Jewish Women's Archive, "Alphabet of Ben Sira 78: Lilith," *Jewish Women's Archive*, jwa.org/node/23210.

2   Gustav Davidson, *A Dictionary of Angels: Including the Fallen Angels* (New York: The Free Press, 1971).

## Conclusion

1   The first American Pluto return began in 2008, when Pluto returned to Capricorn for the first time since the late 1700s. It lasts through 2024. The chart of the United States of America is cast for July 4, 1776, with Pluto at 27 degrees of Capricorn.

# Resources

## Books

*All About Love: New Visions*, bell hooks

*Assuming the Ecosexual Position: The Earth as Lover*, Annie Sprinkle and Beth Stephens, with Jennie Klein

*Body Astrology: A Cosmic Guide to Health, Healing, and Harnessing the Power of the Planets*, Claire Gallagher

*Come As You Are: The Surprising New Science That Will Transform Your Sex Life*, Emily Nagoski, PhD

*Come Together: The Science (and Art!) of Creating Lasting Sexual Connections*, Emily Nagoski, PhD

*Cosmos and Psyche: Intimations of a New World View*, Richard Tarnas

*Fundamentals of Vedic Astrology: Vedic Astrologer's Handbook Vol. 1*, Bepin Behari

*Hot and Unbothered: How to Think About, Talk About, and Have the Sex You Really Want*, Yana Tallon-Hicks

*Mating in Captivity: Reconciling the Erotic and the Domestic*, Esther Perel

*Perv: The Sexual Deviant in All of Us*, Jesse Bering

*Pleasure Activism: The Politics of Feeling Good*, adrienne maree brown

*Postcolonial Astrology: Reading the Planets through Capital, Power, and Labor*, Alice Sparkly Kat

*Queer Cosmos: The Astrology of Queer Identities and Relationships*, Colin Bedell

*Sex For One: The Joy of Selfloving*, Betty Dodson

*The Complete Guide to Living by the Moon: A Holistic Approach to Lunar-Inspired Wellness*, Stephanie Gailing

*The Ethical Slut: A Practical Guide to Polyamory, Open Relationships, and Other Adventures*, Janet W. Hardy and Dossie Easton

*The Inner Sky: How to Make Wiser Choices for a More Fulfilling Life*, Steven Forrest

*The Invisible Orientation: An Introduction to Asexuality*, Julie Sondra Decker

*The Lunar Gospel: The Complete Guide to Your Astrological Moon*, Cal Garrison

*The People's Book of Human Sexuality: Expanding the Sexology Archive*, edited by Bianca I. Laureano

*Urban Tantra: Sacred Sex for the Twenty-First Century*, Barbara Carellas

*Venus and Jupiter: Bridging the Ideal and the Real*, Erin Sullivan

*Visionary Activist Astrology: Become a Secret Agent for Transformation*, Caroline W. Casey

*Why Good Sex Matters: Understanding the Neuroscience of Pleasure for a Smarter, Happier, and More Purpose-Filled Life*, Nan Wise, PhD

*With Pleasure: Managing Trauma Triggers for More Vibrant Sex and Relationships*, August McLaughlin and Jamila Dawson, LMFT

*You Were Born for This: Astrology for Radical Self-Acceptance*, Chani Nicholas

## Podcasts

*Embodied Astrology with Renee Stills*

*Embodiment for the Rest of Us*, Chavonne McClay and Jenn Jackson

*Sex and Psychology Podcast*, Dr. Justin Lehmiller

*Sex with Emily*, Dr. Emily Morse

*Shameless Sex*, Amy Baldwin and April Lampert

*The Astrology Podcast*, Chris Brennan

*Where Should We Begin? with Esther Perel*

## Websites and Apps

astro.com

astro-seek.com

cafeastrology.com

CHANI app

TimePassages app

Astro Gold app

## Inclusive, Diverse, Disability-Friendly Sex Tech and Toy Brands

Cute Little Fuckers

Dame

GetBumpn.com

Hot Octopuss

Liberator (pillows and sex furniture)

## Erotica and Ethical Porn
## (Also Called Feminist Porn)

Dipsea (audio)

Erica Lust films

MakeLoveNotPorn

Pinklabel.tv

Sssh

Quinn (audio)

## Where to Find a Qualified Sex
## Coach or Sex Therapist

ASSECT—The American Association of Sex Educators, Counselors, and Therapists

SSTAR—Society for Sex Therapy and Research

WASC—World Association for Sex Coaches

## Where to Find a Qualified
## Professional Astrologer

OPA—Organization for Professional Astrology

ISAR—International Society for Astrological Research

NCGR—National Council for Geocosmic Research

# Index